The *Spiritual*
Quest *and*
the
Way
of
Yoga

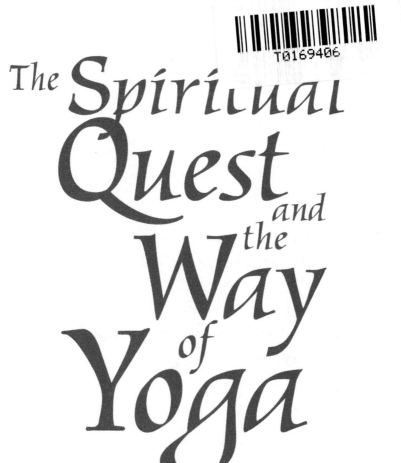

Other books with the Ramakrishna-Vivekananda Center:

Meditation and Its Practices: A Definitive Guide to Techniques and Traditions of Meditation in Yoga and Vedanta

Sri Ramakrishna, the Face of Silence

Sri Sarada Devi, The Holy Mother: Her Teachings and Conversations

The Vedanta Way to Peace and Happiness

The Spiritual Quest and the Way of Yoga

The Goal, the Journey and the Milestones

Swami Adiswarananda

Minister and Spiritual Leader of the
Ramakrishna-Vivekananda Center of New York
and author of *The Vedanta Way to Peace and Happiness*

RAMAKRISHNA-VIVEKANANDA
CENTER OF NEW YORK
"As Many Faiths, So Many Paths"
www.ramakrishna.org

Walking Together, Finding the Way
SKYLIGHT PATHS®
PUBLISHING
Nashville, Tennessee

www.skylightpaths.com

The Spiritual Quest and the Way of Yoga:
The Goal, the Journey and the Milestones

Library of Congress Cataloging-in-Publication Data
Adiswarananda, Swami, 1925–
The spiritual quest and the way of yoga : the goal, the journey and the mile-stones / Swami Adiswarananda.
    p. cm.
ISBN 1-59473-113-6 (hardcover)
1. Yoga. 2. Spiritual life. 3. Vedanta. I. Title.

B132.Y6A36 2005
294.5'4—dc22

2005014078

10 9 8 7 6 5 4 3 2
Manufactured in the United States of America
Cover Design: Sara Dismukes

SkyLight Paths Publishing is creating a place where people of different spiritual traditions come together for challenge and inspiration, a place where we can help each other understand the mystery that lies at the heart of our existence. SkyLight Paths sees both believers and seekers as a community that increasingly transcends traditional boundaries of religion and denomination—people wanting to learn from each other, *walking together, finding the way.*

SkyLight Paths, "Walking Together, Finding the Way," and colophon are trademarks of LongHill Partners, Inc., registered in the U.S. Patent and Trademark Office.

Walking Together, Finding the Way
Published by SkyLight Paths Publishing
A Division of LongHill Partners, Inc.
An Imprint of Turner Publishing Company
4507 Charlotte Avenue, Suite 100
Nashville, TN 37209
Tel: (615) 255-2665
www.skylightpaths.com

Contents

Introduction

There are three basic desires in every human heart: everlasting life, unrestricted awareness, and unbounded joy. All human struggles and efforts are a search for the fulfillment of these three desires. The yoga* philosophy tells us that the fulfillment of these three desires can never become a reality until we discover our true Self, also known as Atman, the divine Self, or God. This true Self is the great Self of the universe and also the inmost Self of all beings and things. It is the Reality of all realities. Only by realizing this Self can a mortal go beyond all sorrow, pain, and suffering. The Self is the source of all bliss and joy. One who has tasted the bliss of the Self never again hankers after anything worldly. This Self, our true identity, is indestructible, eternal, and immortal. One who knows the Self knows everything.

Yet a human individual first seeks the fulfillment of the three desires in the outside world—in holy sanctuaries, places of pilgrimage, and through ascetic renunciation or sense enjoyments. But nowhere does the seeker find that fulfillment. After experiencing repeated births and deaths, pain and pleasure, and being

---

*The word *yoga* in the present book has been used broadly to include both the Yoga philosophy of Patanjali (Yoga with an uppercase *Y*) and that of the Vedanta interpretation of yoga, where yoga means union with the Divine (yoga with a lowercase *y*).

cheated by false hopes, desires, and temptations, the seeker becomes world-weary and begins to look within. This is the first stage of the spiritual quest.

The spiritual quest begins with an awakening to the fact that the sense-perceived world of fleeting enjoyments is the abode of sorrow—where everything is uncertain and where a person finds nobody to call his or her own. The seeker feels intensely restless for the vision of Reality and struggles hard to reach that Reality.

The spiritual quest, from the point of view of yoga, is an inward journey—a journey through the layers of our mind, through the wilderness of temptations, desires, and delusions. The journey has its peaks and valleys, hopes and despairs. The journey is a solitary one, and the seeker's only companion is his or her own mind, known for its proverbial instability and restlessness. The seeker is required to train and educate the mind, distinguish between the facts and myths of life, and prepare for facing temporary setbacks common on the path. The yoga scriptures give us signposts on the path, by which we can judge our progress toward the goal. The Bhagavad Gita tells us that yoga puts an end to all sorrows of life when it is rightly practiced, and practice becomes right when it is steadfast, unbroken, and sincere. Yoga is both light and fire. Before it brings enlightenment, it burns everything false and imaginary. All our desires, enchantments, delusions, and attachments are consumed by that fire. Yoga is raising the blaze of Self-awareness.

In search of self-fulfillment, the seeker turns the mind inward and dives deep within. He or she leaves the sense-perceived world behind, goes through the different layers of attachment to the body, mind, and ego and finally reaches the blissful, immortal, and inmost Self, the focus of the all-pervading universal Self. By tasting the intense bliss of the divine Self, the seeker then becomes absorbed into the Self. Yoga and Vedanta describe this absorption as *samadhi*. The seeker then surfaces to the world of outer consciousness, bringing the great news that the Self alone is the Reality of all realities, the Truth of all truths, and that the Self alone exists in the universe.

The Bhagavad Gita refers to the seeker as a *yogi*, the quest for the Self as *yoga*, the divine Self as *yogeshwara* (the lord of yoga), things necessary to succeed in the quest as *yogakshema*, and assures us that all that is necessary for the quest is the sincere spiritual longing of the seeker for the goal. Everything else comes as a result of divine grace. Reaching the goal and tasting the bliss of the divine Self, the seeker becomes completely transformed, and his or her human birth achieves its highest reward.

The present book explores various aspects of the spiritual quest and answers the question of why a seeker should undertake this quest. Part 1 discusses theories of creation and the meaning of spiritual quest. Part 2 describes the nature of the journey to the goal, the laws of the spiritual highway, and preparations necessary for the journey. Part 3 outlines the milestones of progress, presents a number of vital spiritual questions and their answers, discusses the lessons of history, and summarizes the essential teachings of yoga. The three parts of the book highlight the message of the yoga way: that all the pain and suffering of life are merely the symptoms of a deep-rooted malady that is spiritual. We suffer because of the loss of contact with the center of our being, our true Self. Since the problem is essentially spiritual, it requires a spiritual solution, which is Self-knowledge. Self-knowledge is the goal of all goals, and the quest for Self-knowledge is the greatest of all quests. No attempt in this quest for the Self is ever lost. In the Bhagavad Gita, Arjuna asks Sri Krishna about the ultimate destiny of those who fail to achieve perfection in yoga and realize the Self. To this, Sri Krishna replies:

O Partha, there is no destruction for him either in this world or the next: no evil, My son, befalls a man who does good.

The man who has fallen away from yoga goes to the worlds of the righteous. Having lived there for unnumbered years, he is reborn in the home of the pure and the prosperous.

Or he is born in a family of yogis rich in wisdom. Verily, such a birth is hard to gain in this world.

There he comes in touch with the knowledge acquired in his former body, O son of the Kurus, and strives still further for perfection. (6.40–43)

The yoga way maintains that the spiritual quest is not a matter of choice for us; it is a vital necessity for our total well-being. Self-knowledge, the goal of spiritual quest, is real, tangible, attainable, and verifiable. The yoga way to the Self is direct, well charted, well tested, and its conclusions are based on universal principles. The sages of yoga warn us that those who ignore or neglect this Self become lost in the world of delusion and face the same Self as the unforgiving realities of sorrow and suffering. Only Self-knowledge can save a human individual from the great terrors of life and guarantee everlasting peace.

Many have made painstaking efforts to prepare and edit this book. I am thankful to all of them for their help. I especially thank Mr. Jon Sweeney, the co-founder and former editor in chief of SkyLight Paths Publishing, for his editorial suggestions.

PART ONE

The Goal

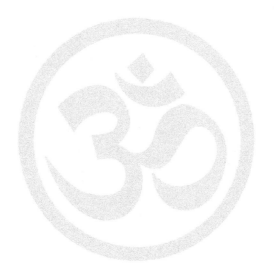

1

Theories of Creation

The spiritual quest is essentially the quest for our self-identity, which is our true Self or soul, worshipped by different traditions through different names and forms. This true Self is the Self of the universe as well as the inmost Self of all beings. The spiritual seeker who makes this quest is called upon to discover and realize that he or she is ultimately connected in every possible way to the universe and that his or her well-being—physical, mental, and spiritual—depends upon the well-being of all in the universe.

The cosmology of different spiritual traditions gives us interpretations of the relative universe around us, the place of the human individual in this universe, and the goal of human life. Any such interpretation is only a working hypothesis for the seeker on the spiritual path. Yet, knowledge of the world and its creation must lead to knowledge of Ultimate Reality, without which all speculations and interpretations of creation are meaningless. Peace and blessedness, the two great rewards of the spiritual quest, can only be attained through knowledge of the Self—not simply through knowledge of the universe around us.

For the spiritual seeker, the cosmology of a particular tradition describes how, why, and when the universe came into being and why the spiritual quest is so important for our well-being.

These questions must be asked and answered in order to understand the meaning of the spiritual quest. This chapter presents various theories that explain the nature of the universe, its origin, and its destiny. According to the traditions of Yoga and Vedanta, all theories of creation come under ten broad categories:

Materialism

Creation as real-unreal

Pluralistic realism

Non-origination of the universe

Momentariness or impermanence

Creation as a combination of atoms and souls

Evolution and involution of nature

Absolute beginning

Transformation of the Divine

Illusory superimposition

MATERIALISM: *SVABHAVA VADA*

The theory of *Svabhava vada* presents a mechanistic and materialistic view of creation. It denies the existence of any conscious purpose behind creation and only believes in observable facts and phenomena. According to this view, the universe of multiplicity is a fortuitous combination of material elements. That which is real is only matter, and consciousness is the evolved form of matter. Such consciousness can emerge out of matter when the elements combine properly. What religions call soul is nothing but a conscious living body. Consciousness has no separate existence independent of the body, and the death of the body, according to this view, is the death of the individual. The advocates of this view argue that things placed under new conditions develop characteristics originally absent in them. Therefore,

heaven and hell, the here and hereafter, the testimony of the scriptures, and the philosophy of religious rituals and sacrifices, are
all mere figments of the imagination or idle speculation.

The believers in *Svabhava vada*, known as Charvakas in the
traditions of Hinduism, ridicule the practice of religious rituals
and sacrifices. According to them, if food offered to a departed
soul in a funeral ceremony can appease the departed soul's hunger,
then food served on the ground floor of a house should easily appease the hunger of a person living on the upper floor. Also, if the
priests really believe that animals used in religious sacrifices attain heaven, then they should also sacrifice their old parents to
ensure their attainment of heaven.[1]

A good action, for the Charvakas, is one that leads to the goal
of maximum pleasure. Therefore, those who renounce sense pleasures for the purpose of attaining something spiritual are like fools
who give up eating fish because of the bones. According to the
modern agnostic Robert Ingersoll, the objects of sense enjoyment
alone are real and the pursuit of maximum sense pleasure is the
one goal of a good life. In a memorable exchange, Ingersoll once
told Swami Vivekananda, the messenger of Vedanta to the West,
"I believe in making the most of this world, in squeezing the or-
ange dry, because this world is all we are sure of."

The swami replied:

> I know a better way to squeeze the orange of this world than
> you do, and I get more out of it. I know I cannot die, so I am
> not in a hurry. I know that there is no fear, so I enjoy the
> squeezing. I have no duty, no bondage of wife and children
> and property, so I can love all men and women. Everyone is
> God to me. Think of the joy of loving man as God! Squeeze
> your orange my way, and you will get every single drop![2]

Svabhava vada is the doctrine of atheism and is really no cosmological doctrine at all. To regard sense pleasure as the only
goal of human life is to abolish all distinction between human

beings and animals. If death were the end of everything, there would be no meaning to life. If the existence of the soul surviving death cannot be demonstrated, neither can its nonexistence and non-survival be proved. The process of creation as an accidental combination of inert matter does not explain any cosmology but rather explains it away. The argument that observable phenomena are the only reality is devoid of any merit, for many such observable phenomena of nature are not true even though they appear to be so. The outlook of *Svabhava vada* is dark and pessimistic. It is really a doctrine of material fatalism.

CREATION AS REAL-UNREAL: *SADASATKARYA VADA*

Sadasatkarya vada is the cosmological theory of "real-unreal." It is supported by Jainism as *Sydvada* and subscribed to by a section of the Mimamsa system of Hinduism as *Svatahpramana vada*.

Sadasatkarya vada describes everything as relative phenomena. That which is real is at the same time unreal: that which is eternal is also ephemeral; and what is true is also imaginary. The doctrine maintains that the world exists only from the point of view of its own substance, space, time, and form, and not from the point of view of others. The reality is, therefore, the totality of all subjective, relative phenomena. It admits the existence of all attributes and all opposite attributes as well, since an absolute affirmation or negation about reality is impossible to establish. The universe is comprised of two eternal, unrelated but coexisting categories: conscious spirit (living souls), and unconscious non-spirit (inert matter).

Sadasatkarya vada believes in rebirth and the law of karma. It rejects the hypothesis that God or any other supernatural authority is responsible for the process of creation. The law of karma alone is responsible. The entire world process is a modification of matter: our body and mind and all other objects are mere combinations of matter. The one unchanging, indivisible substance is time. It cannot be said that everything is fleeting and impermanent; it cannot be said that change is illusory and unreal or that there is a reality that is unchanging. Each living being has a soul that is conscious, and this consciousness is an essential property of the soul. The bondage of the soul is accidental. It is due to wrong identification with the body and mind, both of which are material and subject to the law of karma. Liberation is complete dissociation from matter. It is attained by right knowledge acquired when the results of all karma are exhausted.

This view rules out belief in God or in any other eternally perfect being as the ruler of the universe, since the existence of God cannot be perceived or established through reasoning. It opposes the theory that a world manifesting a design must have a designer, or God. The world cannot be a product of God because an imperceptible, bodiless God cannot produce a concrete and perceptible world. The view also rejects the idea that God is omnipotent and the cause of all beings and things, since practical experience shows us that many objects, such as buildings, houses, and clothes, are not produced by God. It cannot be proved that God is the one and only cause of everything, or that the existence of many gods as causal agents necessarily precludes the possibility of a harmonious universe. The presence of harmony and design need not lead one to posit the existence of God as the grand designer or conductor, since groups of human beings and animals are known to work together in harmony.

Furthermore, the idea of God as an eternal, perfect being is meaningless. Perfection indicates only the removal of imperfection, and it is meaningless to call a being perfect who was never imperfect. According to Jainism, a free soul possessing God-like perfection takes the place of God. Such a soul is called, in human terms, a *jina* or a "victor" and a *vira* or a "hero."

The critics say that *Sadasatkarya vada* seeks to combine the real and existent with the unreal and nonexistent into one category called *the universe* and to declare that both are equally true at the same time. If the theory tries to assert the reality of the partial truth of relative phenomena while denying a view of the absolute, truth would prove partial and incomplete, making *Sadasatkarya vada* itself partially true and partially false.[3] If one rejects the absolute point of view, one must also reject the relative.

Sadasatkarya vada also says that all souls are essentially pure and perfect yet remain separate from each other even after they attain perfection. Likewise, all material elements, even when reduced to one category, are considered qualitatively alike, though separate from one another. This position, however, points out the qualitative unity of all souls and matter while still holding fast to the theory of quantitative diversity of souls and matter. It comes close to describing the unity of spirit and matter but fails to explain how this unity is possible. If all souls are essentially perfect in knowledge, how can they become ignorant?

According to the critics, the claim of joining together various phenomena is an indirect admission of the necessity of an Absolute. Without the unity of the Absolute, there can be no relative phenomena—not to speak of their integration.

PLURALISTIC REALISM: *SVATAHPRAMANA VADA*

Svatahpramana vada is the theory of pluralistic realism as advocated by a section of the Mimamsa system of Hindu philosophy. According to *Svatahpramana vada,* the universe is real, and its reality is self-evident. It is made up of an infinite number of living souls, nonliving atoms, and other material substances. The universe as a whole remains constant and infinite even though a finite number of individual souls and matter come and go. The world process is maintained by the autonomous law of karma and not by any extra-cosmic or supernatural being. Souls are essentially pure substance and devoid of any consciousness. They manifest consciousness only when, due to the law of karma, they assume a body and mind, which are subject to birth, subsistence, growth, maturity, decay, and dissolution. Suffering, according to this doctrine, originates from the association and identification of the soul with the body and mind; cessation from suffering is a result of liberation, which is freedom from all experiences, painful and pleasurable.

Svatahpramana vada emphasizes the law of karma. Karma, or action, produces two kinds of results: immediate (gain or loss) and ultimate (merit or demerit). Good actions produce merit and happiness. Bad actions produce demerit and suffering. The classification of actions into good and bad is in accordance with the injunctions of the Vedas. Only actions such as prayer, worship, charity, austerity, and the fulfilling of vows, when performed in the proper ritualistic way, are regarded as good, because they produce merit. Actions not in accord with the Vedas are considered evil and lead to bondage and suffering. The *Katha Upanishad* says:

> The good is one thing; the pleasant, another. Both of these, serving different needs, bind a man. It goes well with him who, of the two, takes the good; but he who chooses the pleasant misses the end.

> Both the good and the pleasant present themselves to a man. The calm soul examines them well and discriminates. Yea, he prefers the good to the pleasant; but the fool chooses the pleasant out of greed and avarice.[4]

The injunctions of the Vedas, according to this theory, are conducive to the happiness of all because they maintain the moral and social conscience of human life. The doctrine does not postulate the existence of God but instead considers the Vedas as supremely significant. Karma, the performance of actions as prescribed by the Vedas, leads to liberation. Liberating knowledge is attained when the effects of bad actions are overcome through the unselfish performance of one's duties.

The critics say that this theory replaces the authority of God with the injunctions of the Vedas, which it regards as authorless and eternal. The theory lapses into a type of ritualistic mysticism that ignores reason. Shankaracharya comments that a knower of the Self is higher than the Vedas:

> The study of the scriptures is useless so long as the highest Truth is unknown, and it is equally useless when the highest Truth has already been known.

> The scriptures consisting of many words are a dense forest which merely causes the mind to ramble. Hence men of wisdom should earnestly set about knowing the true nature of the Self.

> For one who has been bitten by the serpent of ignorance, the only remedy is the knowledge of Brahman [Ultimate Reality]. Of what avail are the Vedas and (other) scriptures, *mantras* ... and medicines to such a one?[5]

The theory also describes liberating knowledge as a product of right actions. But knowledge is a state of being and cannot be the result of any endeavor. Its classification of actions into good (that is, "religious" actions) and bad (that is, all other actions) is dependent not upon the intent and attitude of the performer but on his or her choice of action and mode of performance. This makes the classification dogmatic.

NON-ORIGINATION OF THE UNIVERSE: *AJATI VADA*

Ajati vada is the theory of non-origination of the universe. It denies both the act and fact of creation. It states that the universe of diverse categories has no existence outside the perceiver's mind. The world is in the mind. The Absolute alone exists. The Absolute is Pure Consciousness, beginningless, changeless, and immortal. It is unborn, uncaused, and incorporeal. The world of diverse categories is make-believe and not real. It is like a mirage in the desert. The mirage is merely an appearance in the mind, while the desert itself is the only reality. The desert can never become the mirage. The

Reality can never become transformed into the elusive universe of multiplicity. That which was nonexistent before and will be nonexistent later is nonexistent in between. That which is real can never produce anything that is illusory and unreal.

> The diversity in the universe does not exist as an entity identical with Atman [the Self], nor does it exist by itself. Neither is it separate from Brahman [Ultimate Reality] nor is it non-separate. This is the statement of the wise.[6]

Ajati vada believes that the various theories of creation are futile attempts to attribute some amount of reality to that which is unreal. Those theories tend to be dogmatic, one-sided, or illogical. According to them, creation is a transformation of God, a manifestation of God's will, an inevitable product of infinite time, or a divine sport for God's own enjoyment. But all attempts to find a beginning of the beginningless, to put a limit on the illimitable, and to describe the indescribable are futile. Gaudapada, the primary proponent of *Ajati vada,* points out that such theories are speculative opinions—not decisive facts.

> The knowers of creation call It creation; the knowers of dissolution, dissolution; and the knowers of preservation, preservation. In truth, all such ideas are always imagined in Atman [the Self].[7]

According to Gaudapada, those who defend the reality of creation behave like children when they accept and are satisfied with relative truth as a substitute for ultimate Truth.

Gaudapada criticizes the view that describes nature as the beginningless cause of which the universe is the effect. According to him, reason cannot prove that the Changeless has become the changing phenomena of the universe and that the Immortal is subject to mortality. If the world of plurality originated from something real and non-dual, it will also be real and non-dual, and there would be no purpose for any human endeavor toward progress.

> How can they who assert that the effect is the cause of the
> cause, and the cause is the cause of the effect, maintain the
> beginninglessness of both cause and effect?

> Those who say that the effect is the cause of the cause and that
> the cause is the cause of the effect maintain, actually, that the
> creation [takes place] after the manner of the birth of father from
> son.

> If causality is asserted, then the order in which cause and ef-
> fect succeed each other must be stated. If it is said that they
> appear simultaneously, then, being like the two horns of an an-
> imal, they cannot be mutually related as cause and effect.[8]

Hence the world is never created, has no beginning, and is not
produced by any cause. Proposing a theory of creation, according to Gaudapada, is as ludicrous and irrelevant as diagnosing
the headache of a headless person.

Gaudapada says that there is essentially no problem, and so
there is no need for a solution.

> There is neither dissolution nor creation, none in bondage and
> none practicing disciplines. There is none seeking Liberation
> and none liberated. This is the absolute truth.[9]

According to Gaudapada, both the problem and solution are
imaginary. The search for a solution is meant for those who believe
that there is a problem. The spiritual quest does not offer us anything new. It only helps to free our mind from all dualistic concepts.

Many critics consider the doctrine of *Ajati vada* radically subjective. The theory, they argue, indirectly upholds solipsism. It altogether ignores the objective aspect of the Absolute and abolishes
distinctions between good and evil and virtue and vice. To consider all relative phenomena as fanciful imaginations existing
only in the mind is subscribing to illusionism—whereas the goal
of the spiritual quest is direct experience of Reality. Some critics
argue that if everything is imaginary, then an imaginary human
being, afflicted by imaginary suffering, resorts to an imaginary

spiritual quest, and attains fulfillment and knowledge that also must be imaginary. This doctrine is regarded by many as life negating and therapeutically useless. It discourages all human ambition and the necessity and reality of the spiritual quest.

MOMENTARINESS OR IMPERMANENCE

This is the theory of creation upheld by Buddhism. According to this theory, there is neither the act of creation nor the fact of creation; the universe is an ongoing process without a maker or a making. The world of beings and things is neither real nor grounded in any reality. All things are relative, conditional, subject to change, and, therefore, momentary—a ceaseless flow of fleeting thoughts and perceptions. "Look upon the world as a bubble: look upon it as a mirage. He who looks thus upon the world, the king of death does not see."[10] A particular being or thing is merely a link in the chain of ceaseless changes. As Heraclitus says:

> In the same river we both step and do not step, we are and are not. It is not possible to step twice into the same river. Upon those that step into the same rivers different and different water flow.[11]

The world is like the flame of a lamp that appears to be one continuous flame, like the appearance of a circle of fire that is actually formed by the whirling of a flaming torch.[12] The sense of continuity is perceived because of the rapidity of successive changes.

The idea of continuity is a vicious circle of cause and effect, giving rise to the ever-repeating condition of birth and rebirth following the law of karma, which does not cease to operate at death. There is no such thing as soul, according to this theory, or any permanent spiritual substance. A person's feeling of individuality is also impermanent. The categories that make up the individual self are its body, feelings, perceptions, desires, subconscious urges, and consciousness, all of which are momentary. That which is born is really produced, and that which is produced must be subject to decay and dissolution and is therefore impermanent:

> That which seems everlasting will perish, that which is high will be laid low; where meeting is, parting will be; where birth is, death will come.[13]

The only reality in the midst of momentariness is suffering. One suffers because one is born; the cause of birth is the desire to be born; the desire to be born arises from attachment to the objects of the world; attachment springs from craving; craving from the thirst for sense pleasure; the thirst for sense pleasure from the dormant urges of the psychophysical organism, which arise from ignorance. Ignorance is the root cause of all suffering.[14] This wheel of cause and effect rotates continuously. Sense desire keeps the wheel rotating. The wheel can be brought to a stop only by reaching the state of desirelessness. Desirelessness dawns in the wake of right knowledge, and right knowledge leads to nirvana. Nirvana literally means blowing out or extinguishing the flame of false individuality that is produced by ignorance and perpetuated by craving for sense enjoyment and clinging to sense experience. Positively, nirvana is bliss; negatively, it is extinguishing the flame of desire. The state of nirvana is neither existence nor nonexistence, neither being nor becoming. It cannot be conceptualized.

Of the many schools of Buddhism, the four well-known ones present different versions of the view of creation. The four schools are the Sunyavadi school, the Yogacarya school, the Sautantrika school, and the Vaibhasika school. The first two schools reflect the views of Mahayana Buddhism and the latter two of Hinayana Buddhism. All four subscribe to the theory of momentariness but disagree on the nature of the unreality of the universe. The nihilistic Sunyavadi school denies reality to everything, whether material or mental. It is all void. According to the Yogacarya school, the school of subjective idealism, that which is real is only mental. The non-mental, material world is devoid of reality. The view is also known as *Vijnana vada*. The upholders of the third view are called Sautantrikas, and they hold that reality is not only of the mind but also of external objects, and the external objects are not perceived but known by inference. The upholders of the fourth school are known as Vaibhasikas. Vaibhasikas, unlike Sautantrikas, hold that the world of objects is directly known through perception and not inferred.

The theory of momentariness or impermanence maintains that the life of a person is an unbroken series of states that are causally connected, just as a lamp burning all day and night is an unbroken series of different flames that are connected causally. Rebirth, according to this view, is not transmigration of the same soul into another body. It is the causation of the next life by the present life. The theory of momentariness is based on the idea of dependent origination and leads to the theory of impermanence. Everything originates from some existing conditions, must change when the conditions change, and is destroyed when the conditions cease to be. This is the universal law.

The theory has been criticized on the following grounds: by negating all ideas about absolute Reality, the theory of momentariness undermines even that which is relative and thus makes everything meaningless; by trying to categorize everything as empirically real, it makes everything ephemeral.

The denial of the existence of any permanent soul is logically inconsistent with its adherence to the law of karma. If the human soul is a bundle of momentary categories, who is it then that performs karma, or actions, and who is it that reaps the results?[15] To accept the law of karma but deny the existence of any doer of actions is like staging a drama without an actor. There cannot be any experience without an experiencer.

Furthermore, if everything were momentary, then bondage and liberation would be impossible. No momentary person would ever feel bound, and no momentary person would ever attain permanent liberation.

By maintaining the view that the individual soul is an aggregate of many moments, the doctrine also caters to a form of nihilism that discourages all human aspirations and achievements. If nothing endures beyond the moment, there can be no meaning to life, no incentive for reaching any spiritual goal such as nirvana. Moreover, the state of nirvana has been described as that of bliss, and this presupposes a conscious identity or soul who can experience such bliss. This identity must be a conscious soul that is permanent and not momentary.

In answer to these criticisms, the advocates of momentariness point out that momentariness does not negate continuity. They maintain that a preceding link in the chain of karma does not become nonexistent until it has given rise to the succeeding link. The cause becomes the effect, and the effect, in turn, becomes a fresh cause to produce a new effect. The succeeding link bears the burden of the preceding one, and this keeps continuity unbroken. The present life of an individual sprouts from its cause—that is, the thoughts, words, and actions of its previous life. The law of karma, according to the upholders of this theory, is the indisputable law of nature. This law pertains to the world of relative phenomena. Like any other law of nature, such as the law of gravitation, it is neither good nor bad but operates without the presence of any conscious agent.

The critics of this theory, however, contend that liberating knowledge is impossible without the presence of a permanent self endowed with a discriminating consciousness that can process all sense perception and cognition and transform them into knowledge, which is an inner realization. The very idea of momentariness implies the presence of an abiding Self, an unchanging witness of the changing phenomena of momentariness.

The theory of momentariness indicates a view of life that is predominantly negative. It is philosophically nihilistic, psychologically pessimistic, and spiritually uninspiring. It repudiates the existence of God and denies the authority of sacred traditions and, in their place, proposes a theory of negative pluralism that is inflated and exaggerated. It views life as suffering; its goal of life, nirvana, is self-extinction; and the way to achieve the goal is world negation.

CREATION AS A COMBINATION OF ATOMS AND SOULS: *NITYAPARAMANUKARANA VADA*

The theory of *Nityaparamanukarana vada* is upheld by the Nyaya and Vaisesika systems of Hindu thought. This theory accepts the fact of creation but not altogether the act of creation. The world of beings and things, it proposes, is made up of the world of souls and the world of atoms. It is a composition and combination of different varieties of atoms—such as those of earth, water, fire, space, time, and mind—and souls. The theory accepts the authority of God—the supreme, omniscient being who rules over the world process—but does not attribute the act of creation to God. God is the efficient cause of the universe but not the material cause. The world of atoms and the world of souls are coeternal and coexistent with God.

This theory upholds the cyclical view of creation: the universe comes into being, endures for a certain length of time, and then dissolves into its basic elements. The process of creation is a reconstruction and reordering of the world of atoms in keeping with the merit and demerit earned by souls in accordance with the law of karma. While the atoms are intrinsically inactive by nature, they become activated to combine and compose a new moral order guided by the will of God and determined by the karma of the souls. Individual souls suffer the miseries of life because they are attached or averse to the results of their actions, which combines the atoms accordingly. The law of karma governs reincarnation. The physical body made up of atomic combinations dissolves in course of time and is replaced by another, subjecting the soul to the pains and pleasures of life according to its karma.

The consciousness of the soul, according to this view, is not its essential nature. The soul acquires consciousness through its association with the body and mind. Consciousness is accidental. The sufferings of the soul come to an end only through liberation that is attained by right knowledge—knowledge that the individual soul is different from and independent of the body and mind. Liberation is the cessation of all experiences, both pleasurable and painful, and also of consciousness, perception, feeling, and knowing. *Nityaparamanukarana vada* claims to be the most realistic of all cosmological theories, since it avoids the extremes and inconsistencies of absolute materialism, absolute theism, subjective idealism, or pure absolutism.

Nityaparamanukarana vada is considered an improvement on the materialistic interpretations of the universe but is not as realistic as it claims. The critics say that it is not a comprehensive synthesis because the unity of the cosmos it envisions is a composite of many distinct parts and categories and not organic and natural.

The theory also limits the authority of God by making God no more than a moral director, eliminating the necessity or possibility of divine grace. The destiny of individual souls is guided by the unrelenting law of karma and not by the will of God. This theory, therefore, is accused of indirectly subscribing to fatalism and predestination.[16]

The critics continue that *Nityaparamanukarana vada* makes the nature of souls appear absurd, because souls are not intrinsically endowed with consciousness. They attain consciousness only when they associate with the body, mind, and the senses. Such an explanation reduces the soul to a nonliving entity.

Liberation, according to this view, is a state of pure substance devoid of all consciousness and experience, which, from a practical point of view, is actually a state of petrification. The souls, as indicated earlier, manifest consciousness only in the state of bondage. The law of karma is inexorable—a law that even God cannot alter. It is said that a Vaishnava saint once mocked the devotionless character of the Vaisesika system by saying, "It is far better to be born even as a jackal in the lovely forest of Vrindavan [the forest of the divine Lord Sri Krishna] than to desire the liberation offered by the Vaisesika."[17]

Shankaracharya repudiates *Nityaparamanukarana vada* by calling it the "semi-destroyer" of the universe. Sri Harsha sarcastically calls it *uluka darshana*. Literally, it means the philosophy of Uluka, another name of Kanada, the founder of the Vaisesika system. But *uluka darshana* could also mean "the philosophy of the owl"—that is to say, a philosophy that seems to be full of wisdom but is in fact nothing more than worship of the material world.[18]

EVOLUTION AND INVOLUTION OF NATURE: *PRAKRITI-PARINAMA VADA*

Prakriti-parinama vada is upheld by the Samkhya and Yoga systems of Hindu thought. The theory accepts the fact of creation but does not attribute this fact to an act of God. It maintains that the reality of the universe is self-evident, and this reality is not a combination of the real and the unreal, nor can it be explained away by signifying it as illusory. Creation, according to this view, is beginningless. It is a cyclical process of the evolution and involution of Prakriti, or nature. Each phase of evolution is preceded by a phase of involution. Each phase of involution is preceded by a phase of evolution. The subtle evolves into the gross, the gross endures for a certain length of time, and then again devolves into the subtle state. These processes are like the outbreathing and inbreathing of a person.

This doctrine views Ultimate Reality not as one but two: Purusha, or Pure Consciousness, and Prakriti, or the world of matter. Purusha is the eternal conscious principle and each living being is also a Purusha. Each Purusha is ever-free, immortal, and incorporeal Pure Consciousness. Purushas are infinite in number, but Prakriti is one, unconscious, and beginningless. The universe cannot originate from the eternal Purusha, since its nature is Pure Consciousness. Prakriti also, being inert and unintelligent matter, cannot itself be the cause of the universe, since it is impossible for conscious individuals, who manifest mind and ego, to emerge from unconscious, inert matter.

The gross, material elements of the universe are diverse and scattered but held together by a unifying force, pointing to a single cause behind the diverse effects. *Prakriti-parinama vada* signifies this cause as Prakriti, or nature. Prakriti cannot evolve into the universe by itself. For it to become active requires the proximity of Purusha. Purusha without Prakriti exists as abstract Pure Consciousness and is therefore "lame." Being unintelligent by nature, Prakriti without Purusha is "blind." Prakriti is the name of the universe of material categories taken in totality. The material universe of nature evolves to serve the purpose of living souls. Life and experience are possible only when Purusha and Prakriti combine: Purusha is the indwelling Pure Consciousness and Prakriti the body, mind, intellect, sense organs, and I-consciousness.

The fabric of Prakriti is made up of the three *gunas* (subtle modes of nature): *sattva* (balance), *rajas* (activity), and *tamas* (inertia). All beings and things of this universe are comprised of these three *gunas,* and all diversities are due to the various combinations of the three. Though ever-free and infinite, Purusha, through its contact with Prakriti, becomes identified with the body, mind, and intellect, and follows the destiny of the material categories of nature (birth, subsistence, growth, maturity, decay, and death) governed by the law of karma.

Prakriti evolves to cater to the needs of each individual Purusha in order to provide experiences that pave the way for its liberation. The Purusha attains liberation only through *viveka-*

jnana, or discriminatory knowledge, by which it realizes its inherent freedom from Prakriti. Liberation is the separation of Purusha from Prakriti. With the awakening of discriminatory knowledge, a Purusha draws its consciousness into itself, and Prakriti ceases to evolve for that Purusha. But Prakriti as a totality continues to remain and evolve for the liberation of other Purushas still desiring the enjoyment and experiences of the material universe.

The evolution of Prakriti is unconscious. Just as a tree unconsciously grows fruit or a magnet attracts iron, Prakriti unconsciously evolves everything for Purusha. The body and mind evolve out of Prakriti not only for the enjoyment of sense objects but also for the attainment of discriminatory knowledge.

Prakriti-parinama vada contends that there is no need for postulating the existence of God or any other supernatural being in order to explain creation. If God created this universe of pain and misery, God would be unjust and cruel. If God's actions are predetermined by the law of karma, God could not be omnipotent.[19] If God were really the embodiment of Pure Consciousness, God could not be the material cause of the universe; the cause of change and mutation characteristic to the creative process could not originate from the unchanging and immutable. The bondage of the Purusha is due to its own self-forgetfulness, and liberation only comes in the wake of Self-knowledge.

Prakriti-parinama vada has been criticized on the grounds of philosophical inconsistencies and unsound logic. The main points of criticism are as follows.

By indicating the world process as an evolution and involution of inert nature, *Prakriti-parinama vada* makes the creation seem somewhat mechanical and magical; the doctrine is therefore only an improved version of the materialistic view of creation as advocated by the atheists.

Prakriti-parinama vada postulates that Ultimate Reality is not one but two: Purusha and Prakriti. If each Purusha is eternal and infinite, and at the same time the number of Purushas is infinite, then the inevitable conclusion is that the number of infinites is infinite, which at best is too abstract, if not unimaginable. The doctrine advocates a type of material non-dualism by reducing all objects into one entity it calls Prakriti, or nature. But at the same time, it subscribes to the view that there are an infinite number of souls—each eternal, immortal, and ever free. That view is a form of pluralism, not non-dualism. By describing Ultimate Reality as consisting of two entities, it postulates two absolutes, which is logically contradictory, creating a disparity between the facts of life, Prakriti, and the real meaning of life, liberation of the Purusha. This disparity is especially obvious when considering the experiences of life. In every experience there are two aspects, the subject and the object, both of which unfold simultaneously. The two, the critics say, are not separate realities as *Prakriti-parinama vada* describes. They are two different aspects of the same reality, and any attempt to separate one from the other makes both of them meaningless. If both Purusha and Prakriti are eternal and independent, there could be no real contact between them, and this precludes any possibility for creation and evolution.[20]

The critics point out that *Prakriti-parinama vada* describes Prakriti as an unintelligent, inert, unconscious reality. But it is difficult to imagine how an unintelligent, inert nature evolves into the manifold universe of beings and things. The objects of the universe do not create themselves but need a conscious agent for their creation. There can be no design without a designer.

The theory also depicts Prakriti as held together by the tension of the three *gunas*. But it is difficult to imagine how a material object, such as a rock, could express the three *gunas* and experience feelings of tranquility, activity, and passivity. Such material objects have shape, size, color, weight, and name, but are devoid of feeling. The three *gunas* cannot be said to possess all the qualities of inert nature. Seeing a landscape, for example, may arouse the feeling of tranquility in one person, restlessness in another, and inertia in still another. It cannot be said, then, that the *gunas* inherently belong to all objects.

Prakriti-parinama vada explains the relationship between the world of souls, Purusha, and the world of matter, Prakriti, as a partnership. Prakriti, by evolving into the manifold world, provides enjoyment and sense experience for Purusha. Two analogies are provided. In the first analogy, Purusha is lame, and Prakriti is blind. The Purusha can see but not walk, and Prakriti can walk but not see—thus the two help each other. The lame Purusha sits on the shoulders of the blind Prakriti, and they move together, guiding each other. This analogy makes both agents appear conscious and active, which is a contradiction of the main assertion that Prakriti is inert and unconscious while Purusha is inactive and the indifferent witness-consciousness. The second analogy compares Purusha to a magnet and Prakriti to iron filings. The Purusha attracts Prakriti. But this again makes the inactive Purusha participate in action.[21]

The theory says that Purusha and Prakriti are by nature diametrically opposed to one another and yet are said to have combined. The critics ask: What is the third entity, the catalyst that brings about the combination? *Prakriti-parinama vada* leaves the question unanswered. However, if it were conceded that Purusha and Prakriti become involved with each other because of the similarities between their natures, once the two distinct entities combined, they could never again be separated; hence, liberation, which is the separation of Purusha from Prakriti, is unachievable.

If both Purusha and Prakriti are independent and eternal, why would Purusha—being the nature of ever-free Pure Consciousness—serve the cause of Prakriti and become subservient to its needs? If it is proposed that Prakriti performs actions while Purusha reaps the results of those actions, it means accepting the idea of vicarious liability. The Purusha will be held responsible for all of the karma performed by Prakriti. But there can be no vicarious liability according to the law of karma.

Prakriti-parinama vada also considers Prakriti unconscious and unintelligent, whose only mission is to provide enjoyment and experience for the Purusha. This is hard to imagine.

The theory also repudiates the existence and authority of God as a creator and preserver of the universe, but endows the unintelligent, unconscious world of matter, Prakriti, with the qualities that can only be attributed to God.

Most importantly, the doctrine describes a state of liberation negative in character: it is emancipation from the bonds of Prakriti; it is cessation of all experiences, pleasurable and painful. This state of liberation is *kaivalya,* or aloneness of the Purusha. *Kaivalya,* the critics say, is a type of withdrawal, taking refuge in isolation without resolving and facing the cause of suffering in a decisive way. Such liberation is more a form of escapism than a state of perfection. It is spiritually uninviting.

ABSOLUTE BEGINNING: *DVAITA VADA*

Dvaita vada is upheld by the dualistic school of Vedanta. It is the cosmological doctrine that subscribes to an unquestioning belief in the absolute power and authority of God, the almighty, supreme, extracosmic person who creates the universe of beings and things by mere will. According to *Dvaita vada,* the universe begins at a certain point in time. It is different from and dependent upon God. The process of creation is a revelation of God— a mystery that defies all logical reasoning and speculation. This theory accepts both the act and fact of creation and invokes the authority of the scriptures to establish the hypotheses—such scriptures being a revelation from God and therefore infallible.[22]

Among the advocates of *Dvaita vada,* some believe that the soul has one term of life; others believe that it reincarnates. All agree, however, that salvation lies in absolute surrender to the will of God. Salvation is eternal life in heaven in constant communion with God. It is the unconditional gift of God and can only be attained through grace. The theory does not recognize any need for speculative reasoning with regard to the questions of how, why, and when the universe was created, since everything is possible for God. Human beings are created in the image of God and suffer miseries by denying God's will. It is said that a famous theologian was once giving a discourse on the story of creation. He was interrupted by a skeptic who asked him what God had been doing before creating heaven and earth; the theologian, visibly annoyed, immediately answered, "Creating hell for the overcurious!"

The critics of this theory, however, regard *Dvaita vada* as dogmatic, because it relies on faith and blind belief and not on reason. The story it proposes makes creation a supernatural event beyond human understanding; therefore, it has no explanation of how evil crept into the creation of a God who is all-good, all-loving, and all-powerful. Moreover, the theory fails to give a reason for all the injustice, inequality, and suffering that occur in the realm of a just and compassionate God. To attribute evil and inequality to the will of God is to make God cruel, unjust, and indifferent to the suffering of his own created beings.

The critics argue that creation is an activity and that activity presupposes an unfulfilled desire. It is logically untenable, they say, to attribute a lack of fulfillment to God, who is the embodiment of all fulfillment and perfection.

It is difficult to imagine how the universe, viewed by this theory as something real and material, can come from nothing. Nor can it be understood how a soul created at a certain point in time can attain eternal life. The everlasting salvation of the faithful after death, as upheld by this theory, is a matter of belief and cannot be verified in life. If salvation is the remedy for the sufferings of life, it must be attainable before death. The problems of earthly life cannot be solved after death. A solution is meaningful only in the context of its problem. The salvation of life, in order to be real, must be experienced while living.

TRANSFORMATION OF THE DIVINE: *BRAHMA-PARINAMA VADA*

Brahma-parinama vada is advocated by the qualified non-dualists of Vedanta. It denies the act of creation but accepts the fact. The fact, according to this theory, is that God, the ultimate and absolute Reality, becomes transformed into the universe of beings and things. As the Lord says in the Bhagavad Gita, "I am the origin of all; from Me all things evolve. The wise know this and worship Me with all their heart."[23] This transformation of the Absolute into diverse relative phenomena is neither apparent nor momentary. It is real and eternal.

The relationship between God and the world of souls is similar to the relationship between the soul and the body. God is the very soul of the universe, and the world of living and nonliving forms is the body of God. God is the soul of nature as well as the soul of all human individuals; both the material and instrumental cause of the universe; immanent in its creation and immanent in its transcendental ground. As Meister Eckhart describes:

> But where is this true possession of God, whereby we really possess him, to be found? This real possession of God is to be found in the heart, in an inner motion of the spirit towards him and striving for him ... Whoever possesses God in their being, has him in a divine manner, and he shines out to them in all things; for them all things taste of God and in all things it is God's image that they see. God is always radiant in them; they are inwardly detached from the world and are in-formed by the loving presence of their God.[24]

God is like a roaring fire, and the diverse categories of the universe are like the sparks emanating from it. God is the sum total of all beings and things, but taken as a totality God transcends the universe. God as absolute Reality is not the abstract, attributeless Pure Consciousness of the non-dualists. God, for the qualified non-dualists, is the Supreme Being, the embodiment of all existence, knowledge, and bliss.[25]

This universe is God's *lila,* or sport, according to *Brahma-parinama vada.* God transforms into the manifold world of beings and things out of pure love—not from any necessity or purpose. All beings and things of the universe are God's playmates. Human beings suffer because they refuse to play their role in life and accept and fulfill God's will. Unable to love God as the embodiment of the totality, the human individual is forced to lead a separative existence, harassed by the pairs of opposites, such as pain and pleasure, birth and death, good and evil. Ignorance of God gives rise to the ego. The ego alienates itself from God and seeks to fulfill its own desires at the cost of what is good for all, the totality of existence. The cessation of suffering lies in liberation from the dictates of the ego. Liberation becomes possible through pure love for God, and the immediate cause of this love is knowledge. The seeker should ask of God: "Lord, what wilt thou have me to do?" (Acts 9:6). Liberation is not union with God but constant communion. Such liberation is a gift of God. It is attained only through God's grace after death. Liberation is the supreme realization revealed by pure love, the keynote of this liberation being, "Thy will be done."

Brahma-parinama vada has been criticized by many who contend that the theory of transformation of the absolute Reality into diverse phenomena goes against the very concept of perfection, for that which is Absolute must also be immutable and incorporeal. To think of the Infinite and Changeless divided into two categories—the finite and the Infinite, the immanent and the transcendent—is by definition impossible. If God has become the universe, all beings and things of the universe would be God, which is pantheism; on the other hand, if it is contended that the universe is only a fractional manifestation of God, it means dividing the indivisible. Shankaracharya gives the example that one cannot obtain a live chicken, slaughter it, cook half of the chicken for dinner and keep the other half for laying eggs.[26]

Brahma-parinama vada maintains that all beings and things of the universe are real but not independent. They are dependent on God. But nothing dependent can be real. The real cannot be subservient to any being or thing. In its philosophy, *Brahma-parinama vada* leans toward non-dualism yet, at the same time, clings to dualism. This contradiction cannot be resolved by the analogy of the body and soul either—that is, that God is the soul and all the created beings and things God's body. The body exists for the soul and disintegrates when the soul departs. It logically follows that the body cannot be thought of as having real existence. This same contradiction applies to the analogy of the whole to the parts as well. The parts cannot have a separate existence that is different from the whole. If the universe really makes up the whole body of God, then God must suffer the miseries and adapt to the changes and imperfections of the universe.[27] This is not, however, how *Brahma-parinama vada* describes God, whom it says is the embodiment of absolute existence, knowledge, and bliss.

Furthermore, while *Brahma-parinama vada* indicates God as the absolute Reality, it asserts that the world of matter and the world of souls are also real. It believes that there is an identity of God and an identity of the world that is qualified by a difference between the two, insisting that both ideas are at the same time true. Identity of and difference between two entities, however, cannot exist simultaneously. Light and darkness cannot be both the same thing and opposites.

This theory claims that the cause of suffering is not embodiment—that is, the entrapment of the soul in the body—but ignorance. Yet, it insists that liberation is attained only when the sense of embodiment is shaken off—that is, when the seeker rejects the false belief that his or her infinite soul can ever become trapped in the finite body. Shankaracharya says:

The stupid man thinks he is the body, the book-learned man identifies himself with the mixture of body and soul, while the sage possessed of realization due to discrimination looks upon the eternal Atman [Self] as his Self, and thinks "I am Brahman."[28]

From this and every other point of view, the absolute Reality described by *Brahma-parinama vada* is not really the Absolute but a conditioned Absolute.

ILLUSORY SUPERIMPOSITION: *VIVARTA VADA*

The cosmological theory advocated by non-dualistic Vedanta is known as *Vivarta vada*, the doctrine of illusory superimposition, as explained by Shankaracharya. Non-dualistic Vedanta claims that it presents a cosmology that avoids the extremes of subjective idealism and objective realism. The outlook of this cosmology is in keeping with the demands of reason and objective inquiry and, compared to all other doctrines, is more probable.

Vivarta vada accepts the fact of creation but not the act. None of the other systems of thought that have tried to explain the meaning of creation have been able to present an explanation that establishes its ultimate cause beyond all doubt. The view that God created the universe out of nothing makes nothing the material cause of everything. If God created the universe from preexisting matter, then matter and not God would be the First Cause. If the universe was not created by God but emanated from God, all the categories of the universe would be equal to God. If the universe evolved from matter, then matter would be, as it were, God. If the universe were illusory, God would have to be the cause of the illusion. If the universe was the creation of each individual mind, then each individual would be the totality. Every philosophical speculation that attempts to bring the world of relative existence and the Absolute into any form of causal relationship is bound to end in failure.

Vivarta vada contends that the world of multiplicity is merely an appearance of the Absolute, the one Ultimate Reality. The universe is real only from the relative point of view and not absolutely real.

According to the non-dualistic theory of *Vivarta vada*, Ultimate Reality is one without a second. This Reality, designated as Brahman, is non-dual Pure Consciousness, incorporeal, infinite, and all pervading. All the other realities the human mind can conceive of are mere reflections of the one absolute Reality. They are relative and have no independent existence apart from Brahman, or the Absolute. *Vivarta vada* describes three kinds of reality: the absolutely real, the objectively real, and the reality of dreams and illusions. Among the various theories, some look upon the reality of the universe as a purely objective phenomenon, some as only subjective, some as simultaneously subjective and objective, and some as neither subjective nor objective. Non-dualistic Vedanta contends that reality is both subjective and objective but not at the same time. If one looks at the whole ocean, one cannot see the individual waves; if one looks at the waves, one cannot fathom the whole ocean.

Vivarta vada says that our experiences in the states of waking, dream, and dreamless sleep cannot be labeled absolutely false or illusory. No one can say for certain that the universe we perceive is nonexistent or unreal. Experiences in the waking state are real so long as one remains awake. Dream experiences are real to the dreamer. It also cannot be said that the infinite Brahman is the creator of the universe or that Brahman transformed itself into the finite categories of the universe. Yet, none can deny the reality of the universe. How, then, did the universe originate?

Vivarta vada maintains that the universe was never created. It is an appearance. The universe is what Brahman appears to be to us and not what Brahman really is to itself. Brahman is the essential reality, while the universe is real only from the existential point of view. The existence of anything always remains grounded in its essence. Thus, the reality of all beings and things in the universe has its basis in the absolute Reality, or Brahman. Non-dualistic Vedanta says that that which is real must be real for all time. In this sense, the world we perceive cannot be real, for it is subject to change. The world is bound by time, space, causation, and I-consciousness. It did not exist before. It will not exist afterward. It is an intermediate existence and, therefore, apparent. The infinite cannot be said to be the aggregate of the finite. Even the sum total of all realities of all the finite categories of the universe fails to measure up to the reality of the infinite.

This contention of *Vivarta vada*, however, must answer some demanding questions: How can Brahman, the non-dual Pure Consciousness, appear as the universe of diversities? If Brahman appears to be full of diversities, what is the cause?

In response, *Vivarta vada* presents the theory of maya. The appearance of Brahman as the world is due to maya. Maya is the very power of Brahman. Brahman and maya are like fire and its power to burn or a mirror and its reflection. Brahman and maya as such are inseparable and nondifferent. As an appearance always remains grounded in reality, so maya remains grounded in Brahman and has no existence apart from Brahman. Brahman is like the infinite, fathomless ocean; maya constitutes the countless waves on its surface. Brahman is like a magician and maya the magician's magical power. Maya, as it were, causes the all-pervading Pure Consciousness to appear as the personal God as well as the world of beings and things. Creation is the process of making the absolute Reality, the one without a second, appear diverse. It is the process of attributing becoming to that which is essentially the nature of being. It is like a mirage in the desert or an oil painting of an infinite number of objects. The variety of objects is solely due to name and form.

If Brahman is taken to be the personal God, the universe of name and form is the personal God's disguise. Brahman is everywhere and in everything. Wherever the presence of Brahman is not recognized or felt, it is there that Brahman appears as maya. Maya, when recognized, is Brahman. Shankaracharya describes the phenomenon of creation as maya and says that maya is *anirvachaniya*, or the inscrutable power of Brahman. Maya is a statement of fact—neither real nor unreal nor both. If the world were real, unalterable, and eternal, all human endeavor would be futile, and life would be meaningless. On the other hand, none can say that the universe is unreal because the world is actually perceived by our senses.

Non-dualistic Vedanta, while it advocates *Vivarta vada*, does not claim that philosophical reasoning can give a decisive answer to the question of creation. No one can know a magician by analyzing his magic. None can know Brahman, the absolute Reality, by analyzing the relative universe. What can be said with certainty is that the real can never be unreal, the infinite finite, the timeless time bound, and the immortal mortal. The reality of the manifold is but an appearance, possible only through the inscrutable power of maya. Maya makes unity appear as variety, and variety is the very basis of life. Life is a coming together of imagination and reality. Creation is making one thing appear to take various forms and names. There is no creation where only unity and perfection prevail. The world, at best, can be said to be the playground of the Absolute. Maya allows the play to go on.

Some non-dualistic thinkers contend that Brahman is limited by the medium of the cosmic maya. Brahman appears as the personal God, who is limited by the medium of individual maya as the individual soul. Others believe that Brahman seen through the medium of maya appears as both the personal God and the world of beings and things. Still others believe that the formless, incorporeal, infinite Pure Consciousness, Brahman, can never be limited. To the individual, Brahman appears as diversity because of the conditioning of maya in the individual mind.

Non-dualistic Vedanta considers maya from two points of view: the cosmic and the individual. Maya is the power of

Brahman, and Brahman is the controller of maya. On the other hand, since individuals exist within the realm of maya, they are controlled by it. Maya in its individual aspect is called *avidya*, or ignorance, which not only veils the knowledge of Brahman and the oneness of existence but in their place projects an illusion of separative existence. In reality, there is only one life and one existence. But an individual often imagines himself or herself to be separate from the rest of the universe, which is nothing but the superimposition of the individual mind on the universe. Thus, maya in the form of ignorance is the individual mind. No causal relationship can be established between Brahman and the universe of name and form. Brahman is the absolute Reality of the universe and remains ever the same, regardless of the epithets and attributes that the individual mind superimposes on it. The reality of Brahman is independent of what the individual minds think, feel, or speculate about it.

Vivarta vada assesses the reality of the manifold world by analyzing an individual in all the three states of consciousness: waking, dream, and dreamless sleep, which correspond, respectively, to the gross, subtle, and causal aspects of our existence from the viewpoint of both the macrocosm and the microcosm. Through this analysis, *Vivarta vada* concludes that the macrocosm and microcosm are built on the same plan, show the same pattern, and are constituted by the same stuff. The Vedanta dictum "That thou art" suggests that the essence of "thou" is the same as the essence of "that"—that is, the individual is essentially the same as the totality. The collective gross universe and the gross individual bodies are intrinsically the same, like the forest and the trees that comprise it. The ignorant identify Ultimate Reality with the material things they possess. The materialists are convinced that the pleasures of the body are limitations of Ultimate Reality. The vitalists look upon it as the mind and believe the doubts and hankerings of the mind to be those of the Ultimate. Buddhists deny the very existence of it, and nihilists think of it as void. To the non-dualists, Brahman is the unchanging ground of all the changing phenomena of the universe. The Ultimate appears as the relative. Brahman appears as maya.

According to *Vivarta vada*, while Brahman is devoid of all names, forms, epithets, and attributes, maya, the power of Brahman, is endowed with certain characteristics:

- Maya is the power of Brahman and cannot exist independent of or separated from Brahman.

- From the viewpoint of the microcosm—the individual soul—maya is ignorance, or *avidya*. This ignorance resides in the individual mind, because the waves of ignorance in the mind, like the experiences in a dream, are private to the individual.

- Maya is beginningless—a state of delusion into which a person lapses unconsciously. Though beginningless, maya ceases to exist for the individual with the dawning of the knowledge of Brahman.

- Maya is something positive though not real. It is not merely non-apprehension but also misapprehension of reality.

- Maya cannot be known without the knowledge of Brahman. Our knowledge of the relative universe of time, space, causation, and I-consciousness, which is maya, is never exhaustive but merely a suggestive knowledge subject to change and modification.

- Maya is the superimposition of the conditioned individual mind.[29]

Brahman alone exists and yet appears as the world of individual souls and the world of matter. The theists look upon Ultimate Reality as God with form, while the non-dualists view it as formless Brahman. Multiplicity is perceived by the individual mind due to its conditioning, and this perception is real only so long as it remains conditioned. Brahman appears as God in relation to the world. Multiplicity is real only from the perspective of the separative ego born of ignorance. *Vivarta vada* maintains that ignorance is the cause of all delusion, giving rise to the various sufferings of life. In this sense, ignorance is the First Cause of the universe of multiplicity. Ignorance brings forth the sense of ego, or I-consciousness, that projects a world bound by rigidities and polarities of consciousness manifesting themselves as pairs of opposites, such as pain and pleasure and good and evil. The universe of the individual ego is a private universe, only real to the individual. Identified with the ego, the individual soul projects the body and mind and innumerable sense objects, and experiences birth and rebirth according to the law of karma. The consciousness of the ego is borrowed. It is the reflected consciousness of the Atman—the individual Self or soul—that is Brahman from the point of view of the totality. The ego, caused by ignorance, develops layers of attachment, aversion, and clinging to life, and acts as a pseudo-self for the individual. Cessation of suffering is possible only when ignorance is dispelled by the knowledge of Brahman, by which the individual soul realizes its oneness with everything. Liberation is the spontaneity of this realization.

Non-dualistic Vedanta and true liberation

The materialists seek liberation in sense pleasures and the theists in ascending to heaven after death; for the Nyaya and Vaisesika systems, liberation is the cessation of all suffering; for the Buddhists, it is nirvana, or extinguishing the flame of individuality; for the Jains, it is the perfection of the soul; for the qualified non-dualists, it is communing with God after death; and for the Yoga and Samkhya systems, it is an absolute isolation (*kaivalya*) of the soul from the bonds of Prakriti.

Non-dualistic Vedanta gives the following interpretation of liberation:

• Liberation is the state where the individual soul completely unifies with the Godhead, or Brahman, which leaves behind no trace of individuality, ego, or I-consciousness. According to Hinduism, this is known as *sajujya mukti. Sajujya mukti* is distinguished from the three other varieties of liberation, namely, *salokya mukti,* in which the devotee dwells in the highest heaven with God after death; *samipya mukti,* in which the devotee enjoys the nearness of God; and *sarshti mukti,* in which the devotee attains equal power with God and also God's divine attributes. These latter three varieties of liberation are still dualistic in nature.

- Liberation is *jivanmukti.* It must be attained and experienced while living. All other forms of liberation occur in the hereafter and are matters of belief, not realization.

- Liberation is not liberation from anything but in the midst of everything. The core of this liberation is freedom, not merely enjoyment or the cessation of suffering. It does not consist of going to another realm or heaven or attaining something that we do not already have. It is realizing who we really are.

- Liberation is essentially Self-knowledge. It is a state of positive bliss.

- Liberation is attained through self-effort, self-control, and self-discipline. Ignorance, which the mind superimposes on itself due to its self-indulgence, must be overcome through one's own effort. There is no such thing as vicarious liberation. One who dies in bondage remains bound even after death. Self-knowledge is awakening, illumination, or revelation. It cannot be planned for, scheduled, or achieved through spiritual disciplines, such as penance, austerity, vows, rituals, or charity. Self-discipline purifies the mind. The non-dual Self is revealed as soon as the mind is purified of all superimpositions.

According to non-dualistic Vedanta, liberation is freedom. The liberated soul is known as the free soul. The free soul demonstrates by actions and words the reality of Brahman and the illusory nature of all relative categories, such as names and forms. The free soul recognizes the individual Self to be the same as the universal Self of all beings, regarding the pain and pleasure of others as his or her own. Ever established in the awareness of the one-ness of existence, the free soul feels through all hearts, thinks with all minds, eats through all mouths, and walks with all feet. The free soul is completely free from all desires and attachments, no longer deluded by the notion of individuality. Though active, the free soul is free from all ideas of a doer, of "me" and "mine"; having no possessions or any sense of possessiveness, the free soul is ever contented within. Whether worshipped by the virtuous or tormented by the wicked, the free soul remains undisturbed in his or her inner peace. Shankaracharya describes the free soul as follows:

> The knower of Atman, who wears no outward mark and is unattached to external things, rests on this body without identification, and experiences all sorts of sense-objects as they come, through others' wish, like a child.[30]

The free soul transcends all scriptural injunctions and social conventions and yet is incapable of setting a bad example or doing anything that is not conducive to the welfare of all beings. The free soul is free but not whimsical, spontaneous but not indiscriminate. The virtues of self-control, humility, unselfishness, purity, kindness, compassion, concentration of mind, and meditation, which the free soul practiced to purify the mind, now cling to him or her like so many jewels. Ever inebriated with the bliss of Supreme Brahman, the free soul is an enigma to this ordinary world. In the words of Shankaracharya, the free soul is:

> Sometimes a fool, sometimes a sage, sometimes possessed of regal splendour; sometimes wandering, sometimes behaving like a motionless python [that seldom moves but waits for

food to come to it], sometimes wearing a benignant expression; sometimes honoured, sometimes insulted, sometimes unknown.[31]

Critics of non-dualistic Vedanta

The cosmological theory of *Vivarta vada*, as advocated by non-dualistic Vedanta, has many critics, who have often criticized it in severe terms. Among them, some argue that its contentions are self-contradictory and logically questionable; others denounce the doctrine as a sophisticated abstraction of philosophy that serves no real purpose in life. The validity of the doctrine with its philosophy of non-dualistic Vedanta has been challenged on the following grounds:

The critics say that in its attempt to explain the meaning of creation, *Vivarta vada* actually explains it away. It regards the world of phenomena as illusory and unreal. The picture of Vedanta's Absolute is cold and indifferent to human concerns. It is "a bloodless Absolute dark with the excess of light."[32]

Vivarta vada projects a view of life that caters to world-weariness if not world-negation. It declares everything to be illusory. If this is true, then life itself—its joys and sorrows—is illusory and so is the human individual. How then, the critics ask, can an illusory individual adopt illusory means to reach the real goal of liberation? If everything is illusory, then an illusory individual overcomes his or her illusory sufferings of life by making an illusory spiritual quest and finally attaining a spiritual goal that cannot but be illusory.

Non-dualistic Vedanta claims that the pairs of opposites, such as good and evil, purity and impurity, and light and darkness, are not real but states of mind; there is nothing in the universe that is absolutely good or absolutely evil; everything is relative; Reality is beyond all relative phenomena and categories; our sense of progress is only an illusion; all there is is only change. Such a view of the real and unreal, the critics say, abolishes all distinction between good and evil and thereby leaves a spiritual seeker without an incentive for making moral and ethical progress—the fundamental requirements for spiritual perfection. This is a lofty philosophy, the critics say, advocating low ethics.[33]

Vivarta vada describes the world of phenomena as maya and maintains that maya is inscrutable and indescribable because it is neither real nor unreal. But to think of something as neither real nor unreal is humanly impossible and, practically speaking, absurd.[34] Vedanta says that maya is something positive (a superimposition) though not real. But if maya is positive, it cannot be illusory, cannot be destroyed, and the cause of bondage (maya, or ignorance) would also have to be positive, real, and permanent. Shankaracharya, however, argues back that not infrequently do unreal things appear to be real. An image in a mirror, though unreal, is an exact reflection of a real object. A nightmare is also unreal but can cause the dreamer to tremble with fear and wake up. Imaginary objects become real if the imagination is strong enough. By its stubborn forcefulness, imagination has been known to cause heart attacks or psychological disorders.[35] To the critics, such arguments are farfetched and unsatisfying. Imagination, they say, like ignorance, is always negative. As ignorance is the absence of knowledge, imagination is the absence of reality.

Non-dualistic Vedanta claims that the unreal and illusory maya is responsible for creating the world of phenomena, which is also illusory. To accept this theory would be to concede that illusion and unreality are capable of overpowering the one Reality. Maya has been described as the cause of ignorance and, thereby, bondage. But how does maya originate and what is the locus of maya? *Vivarta vada* of non-dualistic Vedanta proposes only one universal soul for all beings and things, designating it as Brahman or Atman. Brahman, we are told, is non-dual, infinite, absolute Pure Consciousness. Where, then, is maya to originate from? Maya, or ignorance, cannot originate from Brahman, which is undivided Pure Consciousness, nor can it originate from the individual soul, which is also Brahman. Brahman is said to be self-luminous, self-evident, and the nature of pure knowledge. It does not make sense that maya, or ignorance, can inhere in Brahman. To the critics, the very concept of maya is nothing more than a fanciful myth having no basis in rationality whatsoever.

Another criticism asserts that the upholders of non-dualistic Vedanta are unsure about their own theories, for they are not unanimous in their views. Among the non-dualistic Vedantins, some believe that Brahman limited by maya is God and that Brahman limited by *avidya* (ignorance) is the individual soul. Others believe that God is a reflection of Brahman seen through the medium of maya, while the individual soul is a reflection of Brahman in *avidya*. The former believe in limitation while the latter believe in incomplete reflection. The limitation theory makes *avidya* capable of limiting Brahman, the all-pervading Absolute; the reflection theory fails to explain how formless Brahman can be reflected in maya, which is also formless. To avoid these difficulties, some non-dualists suggest a third view: the original Brahman is essentially identical to its image, maya; but this is more a logical abstraction than a rational explanation. A fourth group of non-dualistic thinkers disagrees with all the above theories. They advocate the theory of appearance: God and the individual soul are inscrutable appearances of Brahman. This only goes to show, the critics say, that *Vivarta vada* is in no way a coherent or concrete cosmological doctrine.

Vivarta vada and Vedanta further claim that Brahman is infinite and indefinable, which means that Brahman must also be unknowable and unattainable. Knowledge of Brahman, then, is only possible of Saguna Brahman—Brahman with attributes and qualities—and not of Nirguna Brahman—Brahman devoid of all attributes and qualities. What the non-dualistic Vedantins claim as knowledge of Nirguna Brahman is therefore only knowledge of Saguna Brahman.

The doctrine of *Vivarta vada* is often looked upon by its critics as a mere modification of the Buddhistic doctrines of *Vijnana vada* and *Sunya vada*.* The Buddhistic *Vijnana vada* advocates absolute idealism. The world is ultimately viewed as unreal, mind-made, having no existence independent of our perception of it. Our sense of reality about the world of phenomena is no more certain than our perception of dream objects in the dream state. The world has no creator nor was it ever created. There is neither the fact of creation nor the act of creation. That which is real is neither momentary nor permanent but transcends all dualism of the perceiver and the perceived. The real existence of the world cannot be proved, because the world is in a state of flux. If everything were real, there could be no possibility of change or motion in the world. If everything were unreal, all beings and things would altogether cease to be. All our perceptions of the world are caused by the illusions and fantasies of our mind, and we cannot describe Reality as it exists in itself; therefore, we should give up all such notions of an Absolute.

The proponents of *Vivarta vada* summarily dismiss the criticism that their doctrine is a modification of the above Buddhistic doctrines. They condemn *Vijnana vada* as nothing more than subjectivism and *Sunya vada* as nothing less than nihilism. Shankaracharya compares the study of these Buddhistic doctrines to digging a well in the sand.[36] Vidyaranya defines a Buddhist as one who is confused, deluded, and an expert in futile logic. To the followers of Ramanuja, *Vijnana vada* is an empty dream while *Sunya vada* is a state of delirium.

Despite these bitter accusations, it is hard to deny that there are similarities between Buddhism and Vedanta and that much of the controversy is due to dogmatism of philosophy and reasoning. The only difference between *Sunya vada* of the Buddhists

---

Vivarta vada is also known as *Brahma-vivarta vada*, and *Vijnana vada* and *Sunya vada* are also known as *Vijnana-vivarta vada* and *Sunya-vivarta vada*.

and *Vivarta vada* of Vedanta is one of emphasis. The Buddhists take the word *sunya* to mean "devoid of reality," while the Vedantins define it as "void." *Sunya vada* emphasizes the absolute unreality of all phenomena, whereas Vedanta emphasizes their relative reality. In the same way, both *Vijnana vada* and Vedanta agree that Ultimate Reality is absolute Pure Consciousness but differ in their views of the world. Vedanta emphasizes that the world, although illusory, does have a practical reality, and it thereby distinguishes between the waking and dream states—the former being relatively more real than the latter. *Vijnana vada*, however, altogether dismisses this distinction and emphasizes that the world of phenomena is neither existent, nor nonexistent, nor both. According to *Vijnana vada*, the world is unreal because it is mind-made, while non-dualistic Vedanta believes that it is unreal because it is indescribable.

The Samkhya and Yoga systems argue against Vedanta's claim that the universal soul is one and not many—that this universal soul is the common soul of all. The Samkhya and Yoga systems ask how one can account for the plurality of minds given one common soul. According to Vedanta, then, there ought to be only one ego, one mind, and one intellect: with the liberation of one, all would be liberated; with the birth of one, all would be born; and the death of one would be the death of all.[37]

But perhaps the most controversial part of *Vivarta vada* is its concept of liberation. Vedanta advocates *jivanmukti*, or liberation while living. Liberation is possible only through the realization of the total identity of one's individual consciousness and the universal consciousness, Brahman, attained in the state of *nirvikalpa samadhi*, in which all perceptions of duality and multiplicity cease forever. The knower of Brahman merges in Brahman once and for all and has no notion of his or her separative existence. To the critics, such liberation is more a state of dissolution than of liberation. A meaningful liberation, they say, must be an experience, and there can be no experience without a conscious, individual identity who has that experience.

Vedanta also maintains that the knower of Brahman, after attaining *nirvikalpa samadhi*, never returns to the plane of phenomenal consciousness. If this were true, then how could one establish the validity of this attainment? The advocates of Vedanta say that, generally speaking, a spiritual seeker who attains *nirvikalpa samadhi* does not and cannot return to phenomenal consciousness. His or her body drops off like a dry leaf after remaining in *nirvikalpa samadhi* for twenty-one days. There are, however, extraordinary souls who do return to phenomenal consciousness, and they demonstrate the truth of Brahman and the validity of Self-knowledge. But the critics challenge this statement with three important questions: If some free souls can return to the phenomenal plane after experiencing *nirvikalpa samadhi*, how do they return? Why do they return? And how is it possible for a knower of Brahman to resume his or her personal individuality—to again desire to live in the world of maya, or ignorance?

The reply of Vedanta to the first two questions is that liberated souls who return to the world of phenomena do so in order to fulfill a divine purpose. Their return is possible only through the inscrutable power of maya. But in the opinion of the critics, "inscrutability" is not an answer. It is a resort to a mystification that is as arbitrary as any form of dogmatism. With regard to the third question, Vedanta replies that a free soul continues to perceive duality, feel hunger and thirst, and so on, only until he or she dies a natural death; but all the perceptions and actions of the free soul are effortless. The ignorant see a free soul behaving like an ordinary individual; but the free soul's ego, or I-consciousness, is merely assumed and not real. A free soul's experience of multiplicity is due to the residual momentum of *prarabdha* karma, or past living. This momentum is compared to the motion of a wheel, which continues to turn as long as the impulse that set the wheel in motion lasts. The critics say that this answer would mean that the knowledge of Brahman, which is supposed to destroy all ignorance and therefore the results of all karma, is not enough to destroy the effects of *prarabdha* karma. This makes *prarabdha* karma more powerful than the knowledge of Brahman. It must follow, then, that the experience of *nirvikalpa samadhi* and even *jivanmukti* is not possible. All that is possible to attain in this life is *savikalpa samadhi*, in which state one's I-consciousness remains. *Nirvikalpa samadhi* is something that cannot be attained before death.

In this same regard, the critics say that Vedanta overemphasizes the concern for personal immortality and salvation at the cost of salvation for all. As the doctrine declares, liberation from maya is only for the individual; Vedanta does not believe in collective liberation. When an individual becomes liberated, the world of maya, the world of bondage and suffering, continues to appear real for all others still in ignorance. This overemphasis on personal liberation thus makes the doctrine of *Vivarta vada* narrow and otherworldly in outlook.

Vivarta vada insists that ignorance, which is positive and the root cause of all physical and mental bondage, can only be removed through discriminatory knowledge; yet it fails to elaborate on how this removal of ignorance is possible. Discrimination requires assertion of the will over one's impulses and actions. Individuals, however, often give in to impulses and sense pleasures fully aware that they are gross obsessions; yet they are still powerless to resist them. When the pull of the impulses is too strong, all discrimination fails. Discrimination is too weak an instrument to subdue the unruly and perverted mind that is subject to wrong physical and mental habits. The bondage of the soul, then, the critics say, is a concrete reality and cannot be removed by mere abstract knowledge. Furthermore, since Vedanta claims that both bondage and liberation are equally unreal, the knowledge of Brahman must also be unreal. No real and definite goal can be attained by unreal knowledge.

CONCLUSION

Diverse theories of creation are due to different views of the Ultimate Reality. The face of the Ultimate is ever shrouded in mystery. Believers in time call it Time. Believers in void call it Void. Believers in Pure Consciousness call it Brahman. Believers in matter call it Matter. No one can give finality to the nature of the Ultimate and, therefore, to the cause of the universe. The *Rig Veda* says, "Truth is one: sages call it by various names" (10.114.5). Affirming this Vedic statement, Sri Ramakrishna says, "God is formless and God is with form too, and He is that which transcends both form and formlessness. He alone can say what else He is."[38] This has given rise to the various theories of creation.

Each theory has its own philosophy and arguments to support its view, and such philosophy and arguments cannot be ignored or brushed aside as altogether meaningless. As all descriptions of the Ultimate are speculative, all theories of creation are speculative. The goal of these philosophical speculations is to understand the world around us from the point of view of reason. Each theory takes up, as it were, one aspect of the universal Truth and tries to interpret it according to its own view. Such interpretations always fall short of the actual picture of the universal Truth. Religion insists on faith. But philosophy emphasizes reason. The ultimate experience of Truth may be an act of faith, but its validity is to be judged through reason. So Swami Vivekananda says, "Religion without philosophy runs into superstition; philosophy without religion becomes dry atheism."[39] Regarding Vedanta, Swami Vivekananda's description is as follows:

> There are six schools of philosophy in India that are regarded as orthodox,* and this is because they believe in the Vedas.

---

*The six systems of orthodox Hindu philosophy, as discussed above, are the Samkhya system of Kapila, the Yoga system of Patanjali, the Vaisesika system of Kanada, the Nyaya system of Gautama, the Purva Mimamsa system of Jaimini, and the Vedanta system (or Uttara Mimamsa system) of Vyasa.

Vyasa's philosophy is *par excellence* that of the Upanishads. He wrote in sutra form, that is, in brief algebraic symbols without nominative or verb. This caused so much ambiguity that out of the *Vedanta Sutras* came dualism, qualified non-dualism, and monism, or the "roaring lion of Vedanta"; and all the great commentators of these different schools were at times conscious liars in order to make the texts suit their philosophy.[40]

The picture of Ultimate Reality presented by non-dualistic Vedanta is neither a dogma nor a private experience but a spiritual truth based on both reason and experience. Shankaracharya has employed reason as far as human reason can go to establish the validity of non-dualism without making any concessions to human emotions and sentiments. The philosophy of non-dualism makes room for many conflicting opinions of philosophy and dares to indicate their ultimate synthesis. Vedanta begins with dualism, passes through qualified non-dualism, and ends in absolute non-dualism, affirming the existence of one, all-pervading Reality, which is the Reality of all realities. The goal of spiritual quest is to realize this Reality and discover that the myriad diversities and complexities of creation are bound together by a bond of spiritual unity and harmony.

2

Sri Ramakrishna and the Thinkers of His Time

The yoga way maintains that Self-knowledge is the goal of all goals and priority of all priorities. Unless we know our true Self, we can never know the nature of the universe around us. The outside world is a reflection of what we see within us. Theories of creation are philosophical speculations, and the philosophers are not unanimous in their views. All these speculations and theories try to explain *how* things happen but fail to explain *why* things happen. Only knowledge of the Self can answer this question of why.

The life story of Sri Ramakrishna, the Godman* of nineteenth-century India, is pertinent in understanding the way of yoga and its vital role in guiding our destiny toward the goal of Self-knowledge. Reminding us of the goal, Sri Ramakrishna said:

> First realize God, then think of the creation and other things. ... If you know one you know all. If you put fifty zeros after a one, you have a large sum; but erase the one and nothing remains. It is the one that makes the many. First one, then many. First God, then His creatures and the world.[1]

---

*The terms *Godman* and *Godwoman* as used in this book refer to the great spiritual masters, prophets, and divine incarnations.

SRI RAMAKRISHNA AND HIS MESSAGE

The seers and sages bring to our world the message of truth that they perceive through their unfailing spiritual visions, while the people around them label them abnormal and look upon their visions as absurd. Whether in the field of science or the domain of spirituality, such visionaries are ahead of their time. The ordinary human mind does not like to accept anything out of the ordinary. "Can anything good come out of Nazareth?" asked the people of Jerusalem derisively when they first heard of the revelations of Christ. But truth must prevail. It waits for the right moment to manifest itself, and then the course of history is forever changed.

It is no surprise that Sri Ramakrishna was looked upon by many people of his time as abnormal and insane. The decadent Hindu orthodoxy looked upon the spiritual visions of Sri Ramakrishna as profane while the new reformists regarded him as a mere unlettered temple priest suffering from the maladies of a monomaniac. It is said that if we do not share the insanity of our neighbors, we will be called insane. Sri Ramakrishna's intense God-intoxication appeared excessive even to the many educated people of his time. They had never experienced *samadhi*, or divine communion, or other subtle realities of the spiritual world. People had long forgotten the nature of a God-centered mind and its constant God-intoxication. It was therefore difficult for them to comprehend the depth and breadth of Sri Ramakrishna's new message of God-consciousness, God-realization, and harmony of faiths.

To the old believers, God was either with form or without form. If one religion was true, the others had to be false. But Sri Ramakrishna spoke in a different vein. God, to him, was both with form and formless at the same time. He saw all religions as equally true. Spurning the limits of philosophical speculation and ridding himself of all dogmatic ideas, he could not remain confined to any sect. Controversy and endless argumentation between sects or faiths had no place in the view of Sri Ramakrishna. God is one. His unity is never limited. Immanent in the universe, God also dwells in human beings and, in essence, God and human beings are non-different. Every minute aspect of God's creation is inseparable from every other and is a manifestation of the Divine. All religious differences to Sri Ramakrishna are due to narrowness and dogmatism.

In Sri Ramakrishna's message of spirituality, there was no sin but only error, no darkness but only absence of light. For his harmony of religions, he never asked anyone to accept something new. His only requirement was sincerity of purpose—a Hindu was to be a sincere Hindu, a Christian a sincere Christian, and a Muslim a sincere Muslim. Only by being sincere to our respective faiths can we compose a real harmony of faiths. A symphony sounds perfect only when each individual note is perfectly played.

But this gospel of catholicity and broadness was not of the customary kind, and the people of Sri Ramakrishna's time were not yet ready to receive it. It had to wait for the right moment.

THE SPIRITUAL FERMENT OF THE TIME

Sri Ramakrishna was born in 1836 and passed away in 1886. Although he spent the major part of his life just seven miles from Calcutta, then the capital of British India, few came to know about him during his lifetime. Still fewer truly realized his message. A new sectarianism—agnostic materialism—had been sweeping over India's intellectual class when Sri Ramakrishna was making his way through the lanes and bylanes of Calcutta with his non-sectarian message of unity and harmony. Many orthodox scholars were unaware of the Godman of the century even though he lived so near them. But the process of history follows its own natural course. "Facts are stubborn things," said the philosopher Agassiz, "until they are connected by a general law." Even a known fact must often wait hundreds of years before its true significance is understood. The Pharisees and Sadducees failed to comprehend Christ's great message, although they knew him well. Buddha's message met with the bitterest of denouncements from the so-called orthodox schools of thought. Sri Ramakrishna's message, too, remained undiscovered in his own time.

A message that is destined to change history takes time to take root in the minds of people. Galileo's conclusion that the earth moves around the sun had to wait for a new generation of astronomers for it to be accepted. Einstein's theories revolutionized the study of physics, but the ushering in of that revolution required years until an inspired new generation of scientists came forward. The message of Sri Ramakrishna had to wait for a new generation of spiritual inquirers, dedicated to the great adventure of God-realization, to receive that message and boldly offer the world a sense of hope and the way to truth.

SRI RAMAKRISHNA'S UNIVERSAL VISION

In the history of religions, the life of Sri Ramakrishna is unique. He had no education in science; yet one can find the essential scientific spirit revealed in his life and teachings. Unlike any of his contemporaries of the orthodox school, he did not study the scriptures; yet the conclusions of the scriptures came to be verified by his own experiences and revelations. His practice of different religions was never motivated by a predetermined plan, and his universalism was not a consequence of extensive travel in far-off lands. Had he studied science, future generations would perhaps have doubted his pure devotion to universal Truth. Had he read the scriptures, they would have taken his revelations and his devotion for the Divine Mother as mere imitation. Had there been even the slightest compromise in his principles, his gospel would have lost its power and influence. Whenever his experiences were put to objective testing, they invariably proved to be true. Whenever his revelations were compared to the testimony of the scriptures, people were astonished to find they were orthodox to the core. Doubts, therefore, only burnished his image; disbelief was resolved into the vitality of his message; and the objective verification of his experiences confirmed the stainless purity of his character and genuine love of God.

The experience of ultimate Truth made Sri Ramakrishna sensitive to the most minute psychological facts. The keenness of his observation, coupled with a power and skill of expression, made it possible for him to describe the indescribable with amazing directness and precision. It was Sri Ramakrishna who for the first time explored the vast and unknown realms of the human soul in all its dimensions. Sri Ramakrishna saw what no eye could see, heard what no ear could hear, and discovered what no mind could comprehend. In his search for Truth, he walked alone and was not understood even by the best Hindus of his time. To a world that indulged in chatter and speculation, he brought certainty of faith. Through his life, he demonstrated that God is very much real and can be realized, not through philosophy or logic but through sincerity of purpose. A prophet at home in his spiritual world, Sri Ramakrishna took up the challenge against the harsh realities of the time—the doubts and skepticism of the educated, the jealousy of the religious leaders, and the hollowness of faith of the so-called faithful. The power of his message overcame all obstacles.

Sri Ramakrishna's earthly ministration was extremely brief. He did not take up a personal mission to preach and propagate his message. He remained completely hidden from the public eye. In his silent and profound life, Sri Ramakrishna combined not only the entirety of past spiritual thoughts but also the aspirations of a new future. During his time, the degeneration was great, the doubts were deep, and therefore the realizations were required to be extraordinary. There had been enough argumentation and speculation. The world needed a living example, a decisive demonstration of the spiritual truth in everyday life. No reform movement—social, political, or economic—could salvage the soul. The answer to all agnostic vagueness is the clarity of direct realization.

In Sri Ramakrishna, there was only God. He remained intoxicated in that divine vision. His mind would dive deep in the ocean of divine consciousness to dredge more deeply the realm of bliss, and only at long intervals, out of compassion, would it return to this world of "me" and "mine" in order to teach others. Such God-intoxication rarely allows for preaching, for accepting a position of leadership, or taking up an active mission on earth. For an earthly ministration, one must take a step down from the state of constant God-consciousness. But the silent thoughts of great souls permeate the atmosphere. Sri Ramakrishna's powerful thoughts, simple purity, burning renunciation, and infinite heart filled the atmosphere around him with a spiritual power that transformed and uplifted all who came under its influence.

SRI RAMAKRISHNA AND NOTED PERSONALITIES OF HIS TIME

All great men and women of original thoughts prefer anonymity, and Sri Ramakrishna was no exception. Only after his passing did his influence begin to spread. Yet during the concluding years of his life, he met with many distinguished persons of his time.

Keshab Chandra Sen

Keshab Chandra Sen, the celebrated Brahmo Samaj leader,* met Sri Ramakrishna in 1875. Early in his life, Keshab felt attracted to the teachings of Christ and became increasingly disinterested in popular Hinduism. He introduced Christ to the Brahmo Samaj and thereupon undertook the study of different religions to discover their essential message. About the time he first met Sri Ramakrishna, Keshab was beginning to form the idea of the harmony of religions, the revelation of which he thought to be his divine calling to spread as the *Navavidhan,* or the New Dispensation. Throughout his life, Keshab remained the dedicated leader of the Brahmo Samaj, but as a result of meetings with Sri Ramakrishna, Keshab intensified his own spiritual practices, which deepened his faith in God.

At their first meeting in 1875, Sri Ramakrishna humbly asked Keshab, "People tell me you have seen God; so I have come to hear from you about God." Uttering these words, Sri Ramakrishna passed into a state of *samadhi.* At first, Keshab and his Brahmo followers took this God-intoxication to be a mere feigning, but as the Master† began conversing with them about the blissful and indescribable nature of God, they very soon recognized the high spiritual realization of this uncommon guest. Sri Ramakrishna recounted one of these conversations in particular:

> When I first met Keshab at Jaygopal's garden house, I remarked, "He is the only one who has dropped his tail." At this people laughed. Keshab said to them: "Don't laugh. There must

---

*The Brahmo Samaj is a theistic organization of India, founded by Raja Rammohan Roy in 1828. It played an important role in shaping the course of India's nineteenth-century renaissance. Open to all without distinction of color, creed, caste, nation, or religion, it was originally dedicated to the "worship and adoration of the Eternal, the Unsearchable, the Immutable Being, who is the Author and Preserver of the Universe."

†*The Master* is an honorific name for Sri Ramakrishna.

be some meaning in his words. Let us ask him." Thereupon I said to Keshab: "The tadpole, so long as it has not dropped its tail, lives only in the water. It cannot move about on dry land. But as soon as it drops its tail it hops out on the bank; then it can live both on land and in water. Likewise, as long as a man has not dropped his tail of ignorance, he can live only in the water of the world. But when he drops his tail, that is to say, when he attains the Knowledge of God, then he can roam about as a free soul, or live as a householder if he likes."[2]

After this first meeting, Sri Ramakrishna and Keshab Chandra Sen often visited each other, Sri Ramakrishna traveling to Calcutta or Keshab coming to Dakshineswar.

In many respects the two were poles apart, though an irresistible inner attraction was to make them intimate friends. The Master had realized God as Pure Spirit and Consciousness, but he believed in the various forms of God as well. Keshab, on the other hand, regarded image worship as idolatry and gave allegorical explanations of the Hindu deities. Keshab was an orator and writer of books and magazine articles; Sri Ramakrishna had a horror of lecturing and hardly knew how to write his own name. Keshab's fame spread far and wide, even reaching the distant shores of England; the Master still led a secluded life in the village of Dakshineswar. Keshab emphasized social reforms for India's regeneration; to Sri Ramakrishna God-realization was the only goal of life. Keshab considered himself a disciple of Christ and accepted in a diluted form the Christian sacraments and Trinity; Sri Ramakrishna was the simple child of Kali, the Divine Mother,*

---

*The Divine Mother Kali is a symbol of the Cosmic Power of Brahman, or the Absolute. She is the totality of the universe, a glorious harmony of the pairs of opposites. She deals out death, as she creates and preserves human life. Kali has three eyes, the third being the symbol of Divine Wisdom of the Self and of Ultimate Reality; they strike dismay into the wicked, yet pour out affection for her devotees.

though he too, in a different way, acknowledged Christ's divinity. Keshab was a householder and took a real interest in the welfare of his children, whereas Sri Ramakrishna was a paramahamsa and completely indifferent to the life of the world. Yet, as their acquaintance ripened into friendship, Sri Ramakrishna and Keshab held each other in great love and respect.[3]

The two often felt anxious to see each other if even a few days passed between visits.[4] Keshab regularly brought his Brahmo followers to Dakshineswar to hear Sri Ramakrishna describe his period of intense spiritual practices and direct vision of God. Keshab would sit near Sri Ramakrishna's feet with all the other devotees. On one such occasion Sri Ramakrishna jokingly said, "Keshab, you charm so many people by your lectures; say something to me." With humility, the great orator replied, "Sir, am I to carry coal to New Castle?"[5]

This attraction then developed into a deep intimacy that broadened Keshab's outlook. He was impressed with Sri Ramakrishna's unification of the various ways to reach God—the ways of knowledge, love, renunciation, and selfless activity—and Sri Ramakrishna's explanation that the essential goal is God-consciousness. On one such occasion when Sri Ramakrishna was speaking of the different attitudes of the *jnani* and the *bhakta,* Keshab "listened to these words with wonder in his eyes" and remarked to the Brahmo members, "I have never before heard such a wonderful and beautiful interpretation of jnana and bhakti." He then conversed further with Sri Ramakrishna:

> *Keshab* (to the Master): How long will you hide yourself in this way. I dare say people will be thronging here by and by in great crowds.
>
> *Master* [Sri Ramakrishna]: What are you talking of? I only eat and drink and sing God's name. I know nothing about gathering crowds....

Keshab: All right, sir, I shall gather the crowd. But they all must come to your place.

Master: I am the dust of the dust of everybody's feet. If anyone is gracious enough to come here, he is welcome.

Keshab: Whatever you may say, sir, your advent cannot be in vain.[6]

In fact, it was Keshab Chandra Sen who brought Sri Ramakrishna to the attention of the Calcutta public through his journal. Sri Ramakrishna one day spoke to Keshab about the articles the Brahmo Samaj published about him:

Why do you write about me in your paper? You cannot make a man great by writing about him in books and magazines. If God makes a man great, then everybody knows about him even though he lives in a forest. When flowers bloom in the deep woods, the bees find them, but the flies do not.... The tongue that praises you today will abuse you tomorrow. I don't want name and fame. May I always remain the humblest of the humble and the lowliest of the lowly![7]

On October 27, 1882, Keshab Chandra Sen made arrangements for his disciples to meet Sri Ramakrishna on a steamboat on the Ganges. A large crowd of Brahmo followers gathered to see the holy man of Dakshineswar. Sri Ramakrishna entered the steamer in an abstracted mood. The Brahmo Samaj believed in a God without form but with love and compassion. Sri Ramakrishna had experienced God to be a living reality far from an intellectual conception. Religion, for Sri Ramakrishna, was to be practiced and the goal of God-consciousness to be attained in this very life; all social and worldly pursuits were only so many obstacles to this goal. There were, for Sri Ramakrishna, infinite paths to reach this goal, and no path, if followed faithfully, was false.

Without any prompting or posed question, Sri Ramakrishna began speaking to the Brahmos about the harmony of religions and the devotee's one goal of God-realization:

The Reality is one and the same; the difference is in name and form.

It is like water, called in different languages by different names, such as "jal," "pani," and so forth. There are three or four ghats on a lake. The Hindus, who drink water at one place, call it "jal." The Mussalmans at another place call it "pani." And the English at a third place call it "water." All three denote one and the same thing, the difference being in the name only. In the same way, some address the Reality as "Allah," some as "God," some as "Brahman," some as "Kali," and others by such names as "Rama," "Jesus," "Durga," and "Hari."[8]

On Wednesday, November 28, 1883, Sri Ramakrishna went to visit Keshab for the last time. He was told by one of Keshab's disciples, "Keshab is now an altogether different person. Like you, sir, he talks to the Divine Mother."[9] When Sri Ramakrishna heard this, he went into a divine mood. At this last meeting, the two only talked of God; to the surprise of those present, neither inquired about the other's health. Perhaps at this time, Keshab, speaking with Sri Ramakrishna for the last time, felt free to express his belief in the unity of the Godhead, which Sri Ramakrishna had directly experienced. His faith in Christ and the Divine Mother was one and the same devotion to God. Sri Ramakrishna said, "He who is aware of the father must also think of the mother." Then, in response to Keshab's laughter, asked, "You understand this, don't you?" Keshab replied, "Yes, sir. I do."[10]

Keshab Chandra Sen indicated the uniqueness of the Master's high spirituality. In his room hung a photograph of the Master in *samadhi,* which was in fact taken at Keshab's house. Someone once pointed out this photograph and told Keshab, "Many people say that he [Sri Ramakrishna] is an incarnation of Chaitanya."* Keshab looked at the picture and affirmed, "One

---

*Sri Chaitanya was a prophet born in Bengal, India, in 1485, who emphasized the path of divine love for the realization of God.

doesn't see such *samadhi*. Only men like Christ, Mohammed, and Chaitanya experienced it."[11] It was in this way that some of the followers of Keshab Chandra Sen and members of the Brahmo Samaj came to know about Sri Ramakrishna, although there were a number of Brahmos who considered him a nuisance.[12] Several of Sri Ramakrishna's direct monastic disciples, including Swami Vivekananda, Swami Brahmananda, Swami Shivananda, Swami Saradananda, and Swami Ramakrishnananda, attended the Brahmo Samaj before meeting Sri Ramakrishna.

It could be said that only after his meeting with Keshab did the general public of Calcutta begin to hear of the Master. Keshab and other Brahmo leaders often quoted Sri Ramakrishna in their lectures, and Calcutta newspapers began publishing articles describing the "pure character, words of wisdom and the liberal religious tenets"[13] of Sri Ramakrishna. For his part, the Master made a special effort to encourage the Brahmos in their spiritual disciplines, always reminding them that realization was the one goal of life, and that social reform and other political activities were secondary. Gradually, Keshab Chandra Sen truly realized this message of the Master and made great advancement in his meditation and spiritual practice.

It is certain that Keshab revered Sri Ramakrishna as a great soul; yet Keshab could not fully accept the ideals of Sri Ramakrishna. In his biography *Sri Ramakrishna, the Great Master,* Swami Saradananda wrote:

> Although he was dearly loved by the Master and had many opportunities to see and hear him, it is doubtful whether Keshab, inspired with Western ideas and ideals as he was, understood him perfectly. For, on the one hand, he looked upon the Master as a living embodiment of spirituality.... On the other hand, he was unable to accept fully the Master's saying, "All religions are true—as many faiths, so many paths," and he tried to found a new faith called "The New Dispensation" by picking

out what appeared to him to be the essentials of all religions and rejecting what seemed non-essentials in them. As this faith came into existence shortly after Keshab's acquaintance with the Master, it appears probable that it was a partial acceptance and propagation of the Master's final conclusion regarding the true nature of all religions.[14]

Devendranath Tagore

Sri Ramakrishna also visited Devendranath Tagore, father of the poet Rabindranath Tagore and a leading organizer of the Brahmo Samaj. Devendranath's nobility and stately character were matched by his faith in the Upanishads as the inspired teachings that would rejuvenate the spiritual culture of India. Hearing of his scholarship and saintly character, Sri Ramakrishna said, "Devendra Tagore thinks of God. I should like to see him." When Sri Ramakrishna heard that anyone chanted the name of God sincerely, he wanted to see that person, paying no regard to whether the person was of high or low social position.

Upon their meeting, Sri Ramakrishna found that Devendranath lived a life of both "yoga and bhoga" (spirituality and worldly enjoyment). He expected to find such a respected spiritual personality full of renunciation and humility but noticed in Devendra "a little vanity." "And isn't that natural?" Sri Ramakrishna later remarked. "He had such wealth, such scholarship, such name and fame!"[15] Scholarship and fame never impressed Sri Ramakrishna. He would often say that the scriptures no doubt help one to find the way to realize God, but then "comes the time for action"[16] in order to develop true love of God. Sri Ramakrishna described their meeting some time later:

He [Devendranath] recited some texts from the Vedas. He said, "This universe is like a chandelier and each living being is a light in it." ... I too had a vision like that. I found his words agreed with my vision, and I thought he must be a very great man. I asked him to explain his words. He said: "God has created men to manifest His own glory; otherwise, who could know this universe? Everything becomes dark without the lights in the chandelier. One cannot even see the chandelier itself."

We talked a long time. Devendra was pleased and said to me, "You must come to our Brahmo Samaj festival." "That," I said, "depends on the will of God. You can see the state of my mind. There's no knowing when God will put me into a particular state." Devendra insisted: "No, you must come. But put on your cloth and wear a shawl over your body. Someone might say something unkind about your untidiness, and that would hurt me." "No," I replied, "I cannot promise that. I cannot be a babu [a dandy]." Devendra and Mathur [a devotee of Sri Ramakrishna] laughed.

The very next day Mathur received a letter from Devendra forbidding me to go to the festival. He wrote that it would be ungentlemanly of me not to cover my body with a shawl.[17]

"Thus," Sri Ramakrishna said about Devendranath Tagore, "though he was a *jnani*, yet he was preoccupied with his worldly life."[18] Devendranath Tagore, therefore, could not recognize the greatness of Sri Ramakrishna at the time.

Shivanath Shastri

The other well-known Brahmo leader, Shivanath Shastri, also had a very intimate relationship with Sri Ramakrishna. Sri Ramakrishna thought Shivanath to be a great devotee of God and said he was "soaked in the love of God, like a cheese-cake in syrup."[19] To Shivanath, Sri Ramakrishna was "no longer a *sadhaka* or a devotee but a *Siddha Purusha* (Realized Soul)." Some time later, Shivanath became the general leader of the Brahmo Samaj. Before this, he often visited the Master at

Dakshineswar and received much affection from him; but now he stopped coming. Swami Vivekananda gives an account of Shivanath's absence:

> Questioned at that time about the reason why he had discontinued going to the Master, Acharya Shivanath said, "If I go there frequently, all the others of the Brahmo Samaj will do so in imitation of me and, as a result, the Samaj will collapse."[20]

Shivanath also believed that Sri Ramakrishna's high state of *samadhi* was "a disease (hysteria or epileptic fits) produced by nervous disorder."[21] He told Swami Vivekananda not to visit Sri Ramakrishna anymore, saying, "The Master's Bhavasamadhi, etc., are the results of his nervous weakness and his brain has got deranged on account of his undergoing too much physical hardship."[22] In an indirect reference to Sri Ramakrishna, Shivanath once remarked that "too much thinking about God confounds the brain."[23] Sri Ramakrishna one day raised the topic and said, "Look here, Shivanath, is it true that you call these [referring to his *samadhi*] a disease and say that I become unconscious at that time? Ah! you people have remained all right, although you apply your minds night and day to insentient things like brick, wood, earth, money, etc., and I, who think night and day on Him, whose consciousness makes the whole universe conscious, become unconscious! Where have you borrowed your intellect from?"[24] Shivanath, of course, could say nothing in reply.

Iswar Chandra Vidyasagar

Iswar Chandra Vidyasagar, another great luminary of nineteenth-century Bengal, met Sri Ramakrishna in 1882. Vidyasagar was widely known for his large heart that embraced the poor, the needy, and all God's creatures. Sri Ramakrishna wanted to visit such a compassionate soul. Before their meeting, Vidyasagar asked

M.* one question about Sri Ramakrishna: "Does he wear an ochre cloth?" To this M. answered, "No, sir. He is an unusual person.... He has no outer indication of holiness. But he doesn't know anything except God. Day and night he thinks of God alone."[25]

Sri Ramakrishna and Vidyasagar met on August 5, 1882. The two great personalities exchanged friendly greetings and made jokes, but Sri Ramakrishna quickly turned the conversation to the subject of the nature and knowledge of Brahman.† When Sri Ramakrishna said, "What Brahman is cannot be described. All things in the world—the Vedas, the Puranas, the Tantras, the six systems of philosophy—have been defiled, like food that has been touched by the tongue, for they have been read or uttered by the tongue. Only one thing has not been defiled in this way, and that is Brahman. No one has ever been able to say what Brahman is," Vidyasagar announced to his friends, "Oh! That is a remarkable statement. I have learnt something new today."[26]

Over and over again, Sri Ramakrishna asked Vidyasagar to "go forward" in his spiritual disciplines, for Vidyasagar's philanthropic activities and dependence on knowledge and reason had caused his spiritual attitude toward God to be dry. About him, M. once reported, "I found out that he didn't much care for what the Vaishnavas call emotion or ecstasy."[27] So Sri Ramakrishna advised Vidyasagar:

One must have faith and love.... If a man comes to love God, he need not trouble himself much about these activities.... The activities that you are engaged in are good. It is very good if you can perform them in a selfless spirit, renouncing egotism, giving up the idea that you are the doer. Through such action one develops love and devotion to God, and ultimately realizes Him.... By these philanthropic activities you are really

---

*Mahendra Nath Gupta, the chronicler of *The Gospel of Sri Ramakrishna* and a prominent householder disciple of Sri Ramakrishna.
†The Absolute; the Supreme Reality.

doing good to yourself. If you can do them disinterestedly, your mind will become pure and you will develop love of God. As soon as you have that love you will realize him.[28]

Again, Sri Ramakrishna said, "Through selfless work, love of God grows in the heart. Then, through His grace, one realizes Him in course of time. God can be seen. One can talk to Him as I am talking to you."[29]

After their meeting, Sri Ramakrishna often remembered and spoke about his meeting with Vidyasagar. Some time later when a devotee asked Sri Ramakrishna his impression of Pundit Vidyasagar, he said:

Vidyasagar has both scholarship and charity, but he lacks inner vision. God lies hidden within him. Had he but found it out, his activities would have been reduced; finally they would have stopped altogether. Had he but known that God resides in his heart, his mind would have been directed to God in thought and meditation. Some persons must perform selfless work a long time before they can practice dispassion and direct their minds to the spiritual ideal and at last be absorbed in God.

The activities that Vidyasagar is engaged in are good. Charity is very noble. [But] there is a great difference between daya, compassion, and maya, attachment.[30]

Sri Ramakrishna intimated that Vidyasagar had both *daya* and maya; but he had also told the Pundit, "There is gold buried in your heart...."[31]

Bankim Chandra Chatterjee

Bankim Chandra Chatterjee, the titan literary figure of nineteenth-century Bengal, once came to see Sri Ramakrishna with the intention of judging his spiritual authenticity. A leading representative of the new renaissance, Bankim was unable to fully measure the depth of Sri Ramakrishna's thoughts and experiences. With a smile, Sri Ramakrishna asked him, "Well, what do you say about man's duties?" Bankim also smiled and answered, "If you ask me about them, I should say they are eating, sleeping, and sex-life." These words from one who was supposedly a scholar and author created a great aversion in Sri Ramakrishna. In a sharp tone, the Master replied:

> Eh? You are very saucy! What you do day and night comes out through your mouth. A man belches what he eats. If he eats radish, he belches radish.... A man who has seen God will never say what you have just said. What will a pundit's scholarship profit him if he does not think of God and has no discrimination and renunciation?...
>
> Kites and vultures soar very high indeed, but their gaze is fixed only on the charnel-pit....
>
> Some may say about the devotees: "Day and night these people speak about God. They are crazy; they have lost their heads. But how clever we are! How we enjoy pleasure—money, honour, the senses!" The crow, too, thinks he is a clever bird; but the first thing he does when he wakes up in the early morning is to fill his stomach with nothing but others' filth. Haven't you noticed how he struts about? Very clever indeed![32]

M., who was present during the conversation, writes, "There was dead silence."[33] The Master went on to describe the single-minded devotion of a devotee of God who has given up attachment to worldly things, then tenderly told Bankim, "Please don't take offense at my words." By this time, Bankim must have realized to some degree the genuineness of Sri Ramakrishna and responded, "Sir, I haven't come here to hear sweet things."

Sri Ramakrishna then asked, "Which comes first, 'science' or God? What do you say?" To this Bankim replied, "How can we know God without knowing something of this world? We should first learn from books." With this reply, Bankim echoed the questioning spirit of the time. Sri Ramakrishna's response was immediate: "That's the one cry from all of you. But God comes first and then the creation. After attaining God you can know everything else, if it is necessary."[34]

The pure love and knowledge of Sri Ramakrishna made a deep impression on Bankim's mind. Toward the end of their conversation he asked, "Sir, how can one develop divine love?" Sri Ramakrishna realized that Bankim had become content having attained scholarship and fame. "Let me tell you something," he advised. "What will you gain by floating on the surface? Dive a little under the water. The gems lie deep under the water; so what is the good of throwing your arms and legs about on the surface? A real gem is heavy. It doesn't float; it sinks to the bottom. To get the real gem you must dive deep." Bankim then joked, "Sir, what can we do? We are tied to a cork. It prevents us from diving." Sri Ramakrishna responded, "All sins vanish if one only remembers God. His name breaks the fetters of death. You must dive deep...." And then he sang for Bankim,

> Dive deep, O mind, dive deep in the Ocean of God's Beauty;
> If you descend to the uttermost depths,
> There you will find the gem of Love....[35]

When Bankim was about to take leave of the Master, he humbly remarked to Sri Ramakrishna, "Sir, I am not such an idiot as you may think."[36]

Dr. Mahendralal Sarkar

Dr. Mahendralal Sarkar, the renowned physician of Calcutta and founder of the Association for the Cultivation of Science, became closely associated with Sri Ramakrishna during the final period of the Master's life. As a doctor, he treated the Master very carefully and, after some time, hearing that the devotees bore the expenses of the Master, refused to accept payment for his services "to help you in your good action,"[37] he told the devotees. A staunch advocate of science and reason, Dr. Sarkar medically examined Sri Ramakrishna while Sri Ramakrishna was in *samadhi.* Sri Ramakrishna was staying at Calcutta for the treatment of his illness at the time. In the state of *samadhi,* Sri Ramakrishna's ego, or I-consciousness, would disappear.[38] Dr. Sarkar was one of several doctors who examined Sri Ramakrishna using a stethoscope and other medical instruments and found that the Master's pulse and heartbeat would stop in the state of *samadhi.* Another doctor went even further and touched the Master's eyeball. The doctor "found it insensitive to touch like that of a dead man."[39] Dr. Sarkar was, then, "stupefied and had to admit that science could not throw any light so far on the state of *samadhi.*"[40]

Dr. Sarkar examined Sri Ramakrishna in the mornings but slowly began to stay some time longer—sometimes six to seven hours—to hear Sri Ramakrishna's conversations with the devotees. Typical of the time, Dr. Sarkar first viewed Sri Ramakrishna as superstitious, insane, and even egotistic. He once told the Master, "People call on God when they are faced with a crisis. Is it for the mere fun of it that they say, 'O Lord! Thou, Thou!'? You speak of God because of that trouble in your throat."[41] But Sri Ramakrishna never denounced Dr. Sarkar's strongly held views. Sri Ramakrishna knew that the famous doctor had genuine faith and love for him, for he also brought his son Amrita to see Sri Ramakrishna. Noticing the doctor's transformation, the Master mentioned, "His faith is growing. Is it possible to get rid of egotism altogether? Such scholarship! Such fame! And he has so much money! But he doesn't show disrespect for what I say."[42] Once, when Sri Ramakrishna was about to thank the doctor for taking such care of him, Dr. Sarkar, at once humble and outspoken, interrupted Sri Ramakrishna:

> Well, do you think I spend so much time for your sake only? I have also a personal interest in it. I derive great joy talking with you.... I like you so much, you know, because of your truth. You cannot deviate a hair's breadth in your speech and actions from what you know as true; they, I find elsewhere, say

one thing and do another. I cannot at all put up with that. Don't think I am flattering you. I am not a fellow of that sort.[43]

Sri Ramakrishna and Dr. Sarkar seemed to have a very open and free relationship. One day Dr. Sarkar asked the Master, "But is it ever possible to get rid of all doubts?"[44]

> *Master:* ... It is not easy to get rid of illusion. It lingers even after the attainment of Knowledge. A man dreamt of a tiger. Then he woke up and his dream vanished. But his heart continued to palpitate....
> *Doctor:* These are fine words.
> *Master* (smiling): What kind of words?
> *Doctor:* Fine.
> *Master:* Then give me a "Thank you." [The Master said the words "thank you" in English.]...
> *Doctor:* ... Why should I give that "Thank you" in words?[45]

Dr. Sarkar told Sri Ramakrishna that *samadhi* aggravated his illness and that long spiritual conversations should be avoided since the Master would often go into *samadhi* at the very thought of God. "The illness you are suffering from does not permit the patient to talk with people," he said. "But my case is an exception. You may talk with me when I am here," to which all the devotees laughed.[46]

Dr. Sarkar believed in knowledge and truth alone and considered the devotion of the devotees, and even of Sri Ramakrishna, an empty display. The Master one day told him, "I found that you are a mine of knowledge; but it is all dry knowledge. You have not tasted divine bliss.... If he [referring to the doctor] ever tastes divine bliss, he will see everything, above and below, filled with it. Then he will not say that whatever he says is right and what others say is wrong. Then he will not utter sharp, strong, and pointed words."[47] Sri Ramakrishna introduced him to Narendra, later Swami Vivekananda, who had also studied Western science and philosophy. One afternoon, in a mood of great renunciation and devotion, Narendra sang at the request of Dr. Sarkar. By his singing, the Master went into a spiritual mood and stood up in divine inebriation. Dr. Sarkar also stood up. "Both patient and physician forgot themselves in the spell created by Narendra's music."[48] Sri Ramakrishna asked the doctor why he stood up along with the others:

> *Master:* You have just noticed the effect of divine ecstasy. What does your "science" say about that? Do you think it is a mere hoax?
>
> *Doctor* (to the Master): I must say that this is all natural, when so many people have experienced it. It cannot be a hoax. (*to Narendra*) When you sang the lines,
>
> > *O Mother, make me mad with Thy love!*
> > *What need have I of knowledge or reason?*
>
> I could hardly control myself. I was about to jump to my feet. With great difficulty I suppressed my emotion. I said to myself, "No, I must not display my feelings."
>
> *Master* (with a smile, to the doctor): You are unshakable and motionless, like Mount Sumeru. You are a very deep soul.[49]

Swami Saradananda writes about Dr. Sarkar's relationship with the Master:

> The Master's love for him and his simple sincere behaviour and spiritual nature attracted the doctor towards him, and a sort of reverence was occupying his heart.... He was now regarding not only the Master but also his devotees with a loving eye and became convinced that they had not made of the Master a false idol. But it is not easy to say how he looked upon their profound faith in and great devotion to the Master. It seems that it appeared to him to be a little excessive.... For, in spite of his being a believer in God, he was so deeply influenced by western education that he was unable to understand how

one could worship or pay reverence to a man as Guru or an incarnation of God when one actually saw in him an extraordinary manifestation of divine Power. He was against this attitude only because he could not understand it.[50]

Dr. Sarkar believed in the theory of infinite progress—that each soul, created by God, should strive to progress until it reached the state of perfection. No person, in his opinion, was greater than another. It is for this reason the doctor did not believe in divine incarnations, or in extraordinary, already perfect, souls who come to earth to fulfill a divine purpose. "Incarnation!" he would say, "What is that? To cower before a man who excretes filth! It is absurd."[51] In this regard, Dr. Sarkar believed Sri Ramakrishna to be egotistic—an egotism, he said, that would eventually "ruin" the Master. Of this matter, Sri Ramakrishna laughingly said, "It is not mentioned in his 'science' that God takes human form; so how can he believe it?"[52] The doctor could only go so far as to say, "I have the greatest regard for him as a man."[53] Yet, Sri Ramakrishna had faith in the spiritual development of the doctor: "I shall not have to tell him very much. When the trunk of a tree is cut almost to the other side, the cutter steps aside. A little later the tree falls down of itself."[54] In that hard but sincere heart, Sri Ramakrishna saw a "spiritual substance" that only required "softening."[55]

Thus, many persons came to visit Sri Ramakrishna, but none could fully understand him.

SRI RAMAKRISHNA AND SWAMI VIVEKANANDA

Not until 1881, with the arrival of Narendra was Sri Ramakrishna truly discovered. Perhaps his mission was divinely ordained to unfold in this way. Only another great mind could comprehend the depth of Sri Ramakrishna's spiritual experiences. The complete Sri Ramakrishna could only be recognized and understood by another Sri Ramakrishna. When the young Narendra first visited the Dakshineswar Temple garden, the Godman saw in the face of that young iconoclast the reflection of his own self.

Sri Ramakrishna saw in the rebel Narendra a true person, a spiritual hero who was not content to believe in the beliefs of others, but was determined to experience Truth for himself, who could convince others of the Truth revealed to him, and who was prepared to single-handedly meet the challenges of all old beliefs. A contemplative philosopher or mountain-dwelling holy personality might have found in that rebel spirit an unwelcome disturber of the peace, but Sri Ramakrishna discovered in him a messenger whose torch, once lit from the divine flame, would never be extinguished. Only such an apostle could fathom the entire structure of Sri Ramakrishna's mind—a mind as deep as it was high. Narendra's criticisms of Sri Ramakrishna's experiences were often bitter, and his arguments against them stubborn, but Sri Ramakrishna found pleasure in the turbulent questioning of his disciple. He knew that Narendra would heed his call, setting aside his arguments and agnosticism to deliver his message of harmony to the West and the world.

On Monday, September 11, 1893, Swami Vivekananda addressed an audience of seven thousand at the World's Parliament of Religions in Chicago. He was a delegate of no particular faith, dogma, or sect, but one who spoke for the spiritual uplifting of all humanity. The swami did not condemn or criticize any faith, believing that all religions were equally valuable paths to reach the one goal. But he warned of the dangers that would come if the message of harmony of religions continued to be ignored or neglected:

> Sectarianism, bigotry, and its horrible descendant, fanaticism, have long possessed this beautiful earth. They have filled the earth with violence, drenched it often and often with human blood, destroyed civilization, and sent whole nations to despair. Had it not been for these horrible demons, human so-

ciety would be far more advanced than it is now. But their time is come; and I fervently hope that the bell that tolled this morning in honor of this convention may be the death-knell of all fanaticism, of all persecutions with the sword or with the pen, and of all uncharitable feelings between persons wending their way to the same goal.[56]

These words of interreligious unity spoken by Swami Vivekananda in the West were what his Master had taught him.

The world will not change if all people are converted to Hinduism, Christianity, Judaism, Buddhism, or Islam; but the world will certainly change when people rise above dogmatism and bigotry and make the message of unity and harmony a living reality.

3

Swami Vivekananda: Vedanta East and West

THE MESSAGE OF VEDANTA

Swami Vivekananda is the world teacher who first brought Vedanta to the West. It was the message he delivered at the Parliament of Religions in Chicago in 1893.

Vedanta literally means "end of the Vedas," that is, the final teaching of the Vedas. It is the consummation of the spiritual thoughts of Hinduism. The conclusions of Vedanta are based on universal principles and are applicable to all people of all times. Vedanta reflects the mood and outlook of Eastern spirituality; its echo can be heard in Buddhism, Jainism, Sikhism, theistic Hinduism, and other spiritual traditions of the East.

The way of Vedanta is direct and decisive. Breaking the barriers of traditions and conventions and cutting through the speculations of theology and philosophy, Vedanta leads the individual soul to its inevitable destiny—union with Brahman, the Supreme Soul and Ultimate Reality. It pushes its search for truth as far as human reason can go and seeks to reach the dizzying heights where everything is reduced to Pure Consciousness. Though developed and perfected in the Indo-Gangetic plain, Vedanta cannot be called Indian, just as the law of gravitation cannot be called British.

The view of the Ultimate

Vedanta maintains that Ultimate Reality is one without a second, and designates it by the name Brahman. Brahman is incorporeal, immutable, all-pervading, absolute Pure Consciousness, beyond all names, forms, and attributes. The various names, forms, and epithets of the Divine, such as Shiva, Kali, Vishnu, Jehovah, Allah, and Father in Heaven, are merely superimpositions of individual seekers on Brahman. For the spiritual fulfillment of seekers of truth, the Supreme Brahman assumes various names and forms.

The view of the individual

The individual soul is a focus of the Supreme Brahman. Designated by Vedanta as Atman, it is ever divine and ever pure. Atman is different from the ego-self that is generally assumed to be the soul of a person. A human individual is a layered being whose soul is encased by five sheaths—physical body, vital air, mind, intellect, and bliss. All five sheaths, according to Vedanta, are material. As Swami Vivekananda defines:

> Man, therefore, according to the Vedanta philosophy, is the greatest being in the universe, and this earth the best place in it, because only here is the greatest and the best chance for him to become perfect. Angels or gods, or whatever you may call them, all have to become men if they want to become perfect. This is the great centre, the wonderful opportunity—this human life.[1]

The world view

As discussed in chapter 1, Vedanta subscribes to the view of *Vivarta vada*, according to which the world of myriad diversity is the dynamic manifestation of Brahman in time and space, caused by Brahman's own inscrutable power, known as maya. Maya blocks the view of Brahman and in its place projects a world of diversity; therefore, it is said that the world exists only in the mind of the individual. Good and evil, pain and pleasure, heaven and hell, are all in the individual mind. Nothing in this world is absolutely good or absolutely evil. In a psychological sense, the earth rotates not so much around the sun as around the individual mind.

Maya is not a peculiar concept of Vedanta. The Buddhist tradition calls it *Mara*; the Taoist tradition says it is being "out of harmony with Tao"; the Islamic tradition personifies it as *Iblis*, and the Zoroastrian as *Ahriman*; Platonism refers to it as delusion, and the Judeo-Christian tradition points to sin as a barrier to knowing God. Beings and things in the realm of maya are illusory and ephemeral. They appear real because they reflect the light of the Absolute.

The problem of suffering

The sufferings of life are not due to the retribution of God, to luck, chance, hostile stars or planets, or to any other external agency. Vedanta attributes suffering to five causes: ignorance that brings loss of contact with the Real—the center of our being, the Atman; ego; attachment; aversion; and clinging to life. Loss of contact with the Real forces the individual into the world of ego—a fanciful world of polarization, imagination, and dream. Birth and death, pain and pleasure, here and hereafter, the law of karma and reincarnation, all apply to ego and its world. The decisive way to the end of suffering is to reestablish contact with the Real through Self-knowledge. Swami Vivekananda describes:

> Vedanta says that the cause of all that is apparently evil is the limitation of the Unlimited. The love which gets limited into little channels and seems to be evil eventually comes out at the other end and manifests itself as God. Vedanta also says that the cause of all this apparent evil is in ourselves. Do not blame

any supernatural being; neither be hopeless or despondent, nor think we are in a place from which we can never escape unless someone comes and lends us a helping hand. That cannot be, says Vedanta. We are like silk-worms. We make the thread out of our own substance, and spin the cocoon, and in the course of time are imprisoned inside. But this cannot be for ever. We shall develop spiritual realization in the cocoon and, like the butterfly, come out free. We have woven this network of karma around ourselves, and in our ignorance we feel as if we are bound, and weep and wail for help. But help does not come from without; it comes from within ourselves.[2]

The goal of life

Self-knowledge is the goal of human life. It alone can put an end to our sorrow and suffering. Ignorance, the root cause of all ills, gives rise to ego, which obscures the world of non-dual Reality. Such ignorance can be removed only by knowledge of Reality. Darkness that causes delusive cognition can be removed only by the light of Self-knowledge. Swami Vivekananda says:

> All the strength and succour you want is within yourselves. Therefore make your own future. Let the dead past bury its dead. The infinite future is before you, and you must always remember that each word, thought, and deed lays up a store for you, and that as the bad thoughts and bad works are ready to spring upon you like tigers, so also there is the inspiring hope that the good thoughts and good deeds are ready with the power of a hundred thousand angels to defend you always and for ever.[3]

The quest for immortality

Self-knowledge alone can conquer death. The doctrine of the total annihilation of the soul at the point of death is inconsistent with the desire for immortality innate in every person and against the moral order of the universe. The doctrine that the soul is created at the time of birth and then lives forever lacks a rational basis; it does not satisfactorily explain the fact of inequality between one person and another in physical, mental, moral, and spiritual spheres. The doctrine of eternal happiness in heaven after death goes against logical thinking. Everlasting life in terms of time is irrational. Again, the doctrine of eternal suffering in hell for the mistakes of a few years on earth is contrary to any sense of God's justice and impartial love.

Vedanta says that the individual soul is none other than the Supreme Soul, the Common Soul of all beings, and is immortal. Despite its immortal nature, the individual soul experiences birth and death because of its identification with the body and mind due to ignorance. The experiences of pain and suffering life after life force the soul to ponder the so-called happiness on earth and in heaven and thus spur the soul to practice desirelessness and realize its immortal nature. Self-knowledge is the inescapable destiny of every soul. Through repeated birth and death, each soul, consciously or unconsciously, is moving toward Self-knowledge. Swami Vivekananda describes:

> Picture the embodied self to be the rider and this body the chariot, the intellect to be the charioteer, the mind the reins, and the senses the horses. He whose horses are well broken in and whose reins are strong and kept well in the hands of the charioteer (the intellect) reaches the goal, which is the supreme state of Him, the Omnipresent. But the man whose horses are not controlled, and whose reins are not well managed, goes to destruction.
>
> This Atman, hidden in all beings, does not manifest Itself to the eyes or the senses; but those whose minds have become purified and refined realize It. Beyond all sound and all sight, beyond form, immutable, beyond all taste and touch, infinite, without beginning and without end, even beyond nature,

and unchangeable—he who thus realizes It frees himself from the jaws of death.[4]

The meaning of liberation

Self-knowledge is the liberation of the soul from the bondage of body and mind. It is true awakening—a return to the divinity of one's real Self. Vedanta maintains that there is no liberation without the realization that the individual soul and the Supreme Soul are identical in essence, and this liberation, in order to be true, must be attained before death. Any other form of liberation after death is a matter of faith and speculation. Swami Vivekananda says:

> The Vedanta teaches that Nirvana can be attained here and now, that we do not have to wait for death to reach it. Nirvana is the realisation of the Self; and after having once known that, if only for an instant, never again can one be deluded by the mirage of personality. Having eyes, we must see the apparent, but all the time we know what it is; we have found out its true nature. It is the screen that hides the Self, which is unchanging. The screen opens, and we find the Self behind it. All change is in the screen. In the saint the screen is thin, and the reality can almost shine through. In the sinner the screen is thick, and we are liable to lose sight of the truth that the Atman is there, as well as behind the saint's screen. When the screen is wholly removed, we find it never existed—that we were the Atman and nothing else, even the screen is forgotten.[5]

The knower of Self is called a free soul. Such a person is no longer deluded by appearances. Having realized the oneness of existence, the free soul regards the pleasure and pain of others as his or her own pleasure and pain. The free soul loves all beings and never becomes a cause of fear to anyone. The free soul demonstrates the reality of God and gives validity to the words of the scriptures. The continuance of the body after the attainment of Self-knowledge is not incompatible with liberation.

Four values of life

Vedanta speaks of four values of life: righteous conduct, acquisition of wealth, enjoyment of legitimate pleasures, and Self-knowledge. Righteous conduct is the performance of the duties of life in accordance with the laws of morality and ethics—the foundation of self-development and self-fulfillment. Acquisition of wealth is necessary for the preservation of life and the promotion of the welfare of others. Without the enjoyment of legitimate pleasures, life becomes joyless and dry.

The first three values must find their fulfillment in the fourth, Self-knowledge. Moral perfection when not attained for the sake of Self-knowledge creates enlightened egoism. Wealth and prosperity when not used for the sake of Self-knowledge breed delusion and attachment. Art and aesthetics when they do not reflect the light of the Self degenerate into promiscuity. Knowledge of science and technology when not directed to the attainment of Self-knowledge proves to be a weapon of self-destruction. Self-knowledge is neither an intellectual conviction nor an emotional thrill. It is a burning realization that silences all doubt and transforms a person forever. Self-knowledge is neither miraculous nor is it achieved vicariously. It results from the total response of the whole mind gathered through the practices of self-control and desirelessness.

The four paths to the goal

The way to the liberation of the soul through Self-knowledge is called yoga. Vedanta speaks of four yogas, or paths to the goal: *jnana-yoga,* or the direct way of knowledge; *bhakti-yoga,* or the natural way of divine love; *karma-yoga,* or the practical way of selfless action; and *raja-yoga,* or the scientific way of concentration and meditation. The primary roadblock to Self-knowledge is the restless mind. The four yogas are four ways to overcome the mind's restlessness.

The path of *jnana-yoga* advocates the method of persuasion through reason, saying that only reason can overcome unreason, the cause of all restlessness. *Bhakti-yoga* looks upon the cause of restlessness as the mind's impurity, and prescribes worship, prayer, and self-surrender to the Divine for its purification. *Karma-yoga* views the intoxicated ego as the cause of all restlessness, and calls for eradication of the ego to overcome restlessness. *Raja-yoga* upholds the method of confrontation, maintaining that restlessness of mind has its root deep in the psychophysical system. It holds that reason is too weak to uproot ingrained habits, that worship and prayer require inborn faith in God in order to be effective, and that eradication of the elusive ego is almost impossible. Therefore, *raja-yoga* calls for confronting the restless mind through concentration and meditation and by control of posture and breathing.

To bring the mind under control is the central purpose of all the yoga disciplines. For the spiritual seeker, the ultimate battlefield is the battlefield of the mind. Vedanta maintains that the mind never becomes controlled by itself. It is controlled only through conscious and deliberate effort.

The four cardinal principles

The four cardinal principles of Vedanta are non-duality of the Godhead, divinity of the soul, oneness of existence, and harmony of religions. These are not dogmas, but four universal principles in keeping with reason and everyday personal experience. There is but one Ultimate Reality, and it is described by various names. Furthermore, all religions proclaim that the individual soul is divine. This divinity is innate, not acquired or given; practice of spiritual discipline endows us with faith in our own divinity. Oneness of existence is the foundation for ethics and morality; life is interdependent, not independent. Harmony of religions is the natural corollary to the first three cardinal principles. Different religions are only different pathways to the same goal—God-consciousness. When we move toward this goal voluntarily and consciously, we call it a spiritual quest; when this move is involuntary and forced by nature, we call it an evolutionary process. Vedanta repudiates proselytism, which is a psychologically disruptive and morally reprehensible act.

The harmony of religions is not uniformity. It is unity in diversity. This harmony is not to be attained by mere intellectual understanding and interfaith deliberations, nor can it be enacted by law. It is to be discovered and realized by deepening our individual God-consciousness.

VEDANTA'S CONTRIBUTION TO WORLD THOUGHT

Vedanta's major contribution to world religious thought has been its spiritual democracy, spiritual humanism, and an enduring bond of world unity.

Vedanta fosters spiritual democracy. While other traditions present only one ideal and one path, Vedanta offers an infinite variety of ideals and paths to choose from in order to reach the same ultimate goal. Lacking this freedom of spiritual democracy, religion becomes authoritarian and oppressive, insisting upon blind obedience to rigid traditions and dogmas and unquestioning belief in ceremonials and creeds. Spiritual freedom encourages spiritual individuality, critical inquiry, honest doubt, free choice of the path, and verification of truth through personal experience. The ideas of exclusive salvation, a jealous God, and a chosen people are all alien to Vedanta.

The second major contribution of Vedanta is spiritual humanism, as opposed to secular humanism. Spiritual humanism is not simply doing good to others but rendering loving service to the Divine, seeing its presence in all beings. Spiritual human-ism embraces the whole of humanity, regardless of race, culture, country, religion, or social affiliation.

The third major contribution of Vedanta is its ideal for an en-during bond of world unity. World unity based on political con-siderations, economic interest, cultural ties, or humanitarian principles is never enduring. The bonds of such kinds of unity are too fragile to withstand the stresses and strains of social diversi-ties. Social diversities without spiritual unity become explosive and dangerous to society. Unity of the world body, in order to be real, must be organic—and this requires a world soul that em-braces the countless diversities of human experience and human aspirations. Such a world soul must be the soul of all beings. Vedanta designates that world soul as the all-pervading Self, which is the common Self of both the macrocosm and the mi-crocosm. The unity of this Self includes not only human beings, but also animals, plants, and every form of life.

Critics often perceive this unity as anthropomorphism. Science, however, has proved that consciousness is as much pres-ent in the galaxy as it is in a tiny plant, an animal, or a human being—it is only the manifestation of consciousness that varies. The universe is organically woven. No one can move one atom of the universe without affecting the whole universe. No one can be truly happy by keeping the rest of the world unhappy. No one can live in peace on an island of prosperity surrounded by a sea of poverty and suffering.

Present-day secular culture has broken the unity of existence. It has replaced cooperation with competition and interdepen-dence with the struggle for survival. It has ignored the Socratic teaching that knowledge is virtue and replaced it with its own: knowledge is power. This has set in motion a chain reaction of alienation—from Reality, from nature, and from our true Self. Vedanta seeks to give us back our spiritual connection with all be-ings and things.

THE NINETEENTH-CENTURY ECLIPSE OF VEDANTA

The nineteenth century witnessed an unprecedented spiritual eclipse in India. Vedanta lost its fire and vigor and ceased to be a social reality. That which is the teaching for the strong-minded became a refuge for the weak and the escapists. The philosophy of Vedanta became life negating, not life giving. The spiritual values it championed became separated from the material values that were their support. In search of God in heaven, the Vedantist ignored God in the human heart. Followers of Vedanta forgot that holiness means nothing unless it brings happiness, that filling the empty stomach must come before filling the empty heart, and that renunciation presupposes acquiring and enjoying things to renounce. Passivity became the keynote of Vedanta and self-withdrawal its prime virtue. Inertia passed for tranquility and hopelessness for dispassion.

Vedanta's spiritual quest encouraged a morbid inwardness, a flight from the world in despair over life and its problems. Once a teaching of hope and strength, Vedanta of that time exaggerated human weakness, unworthiness, and sinfulness, focusing only on human limitations and not on human possibilities. Vedanta became a hollow philosophy of life that produced only fake reformers, dreamy idealists, idle philosophers, and so-called knowers of truth who sought transcendental solutions for earthly problems. It created pessimists who proclaimed life intolerable yet continued to tolerate it. Except in the case of a few *sannyasins*, the wisdom of Vedanta was lost in the wilderness of superstition, false piety, eroticism, occultism, and fatalism.

The reasons for the eclipse are obvious. Self-knowledge, the goal of Vedanta, has two aspects: mysticism and humanism. One is seeing God with eyes closed, seeing all in one's Self. The other is seeing the same God with eyes open, seeing one's Self in all. The first without the second is sterile; the second without the first is meaningless. Vedanta of nineteenth-century India tilted too much toward mysticism and lost sight of humanism.

When mysticism and humanism become separated, both degenerate. Mysticism turns into a dreamy search for salvation in a transcendental realm. Humanism without mysticism eventually degenerates into an enlightened egoism obsessed with self-interest. Philanthropy and works of welfare become drab substitutes for spirituality, futile efforts to fill the spiritual void left by the decay of faith. Where there is nothing beyond the present to be hoped for, the philosophy of secular humanism tries to make life less wretched. As the tide of spirituality recedes, the tide of materialism rises. We cease to think of our immortal soul, of the supreme goal of our life, and of the sublime secrets of the universe. This is where Western humanism stands today, having lost its link with mysticism.

SWAMI VIVEKANANDA REVITALIZES VEDANTA

Swami Vivekananda was a synthesis of the cultures of the East and West. As young Narendra, he was daring, quick, full of life, and tempered in the fire of purity and holiness. His keen intellect seized upon the theories and practices of both the Eastern and Western minds but was in a dilemma in an attempt to reconcile faith with reason. The Western readiness to reason its way to truth, its active and often bloody quest for liberty and social justice, fascinated Narendra in his early youth. Yet, in the midst of his intellectual joy, there was a deep longing for God, whose existence could not be proved by reason. The two streams of thought created a terrible commotion within him, and he became a wandering threat to the holy men of his time with his single forthright question: "Sir, have you seen God?"

The search for God ultimately brought Narendra to Sri Ramakrishna, whom, after six years of struggle, he accepted as his teacher. From Sri Ramakrishna he learned the true spirit of

Vedanta. If Narendra reasoned too much and doubted too long it was because his longing for knowledge was too deep and his spiritual hunger was too intense. His contact with the Godman of nineteenth-century India turned the iconoclastic, rebellious young Narendra into a flaming Vivekananda, the very embodiment of Vedanta. One day his dying Master passed onto him his final word of Vedanta—the worship of the living God.

Sri Ramakrishna asked Swami Vivekananda to become like a huge banyan tree, under whose shade would gather weary souls in search of peace and solace in life. After Sri Ramakrishna's passing, Vivekananda set out on a pilgrimage to the shrines of the living God. What Vivekananda saw of India's masses made him restless and brought his mind down from the heights of transcendental consciousness to the misery of the world around him. He saw the land of the all-pervading Brahman filled with cries of sorrow and suffering. The living God in all hearts that Vedanta glorifies was being neglected, insulted, and trampled upon.

Swami Vivekananda became determined to put an end to this insult and neglect of the living God. He decided to awaken the masses by sounding the thundering drumbeats of Vedanta. He saw people in India worshipping "local superstitions" in the name of Vedanta. A proliferation of dogmas, creeds, rituals, and theological speculations obscured the real teachings of Vedanta.

Swami Vivekananda saw India in a deep spiritual coma. He looked toward the West and realized that he needed Western vigor, courage, and tenacity to make Vedanta alive. He wrote that he wished to infuse some of the American spirit into India, into "that awful mass of conservative jelly-fish, and then throw overboard all old associations and start a new thing, entirely new— simple, strong, new, and fresh as the first-born baby—throw all of the past overboard and begin anew."[6]

There is an apparent contradiction between the outlook of the East and that of the West. For the East, knowledge is virtue; it is being as opposed to becoming. For the West, knowledge is not merely virtue but is also a tool to improve the quality of life; knowledge is becoming. Knowledge is the ability to deal with objects in a practical and dynamic way that is capable of changing external nature, accomplishing goals, and bringing about material improvement. The East seeks peace of soul at the price of submission, while the West seeks freedom at the price of bloody combat.

The East is concerned with finding the ultimate solution to the problems of life by absorption in the silence of the Self; it considers the world a mirage, a framework of illusion, maya, a "dog's curly tail" impossible to straighten. Progress, the East says, is illusory, for we live not in a progressive world but in a changing world. To try to build the Kingdom of Heaven on earth is futile. Nothing truly good is to be achieved by material improvement. There is no use trying to make the dog's curly tail straight, to run after the mirage for water. It is foolish to try to save this world of delusion or make it better. Liberation of the soul calls for renunciation of desires—not their multiplication.

The West looks upon these views as pessimistic, otherworldly, and self-defeating. The ultimate goal can never be reached by bypassing immediate needs; one who is not fit for the earth is not fit for heaven. Without material fulfillment, the hope for spiritual attainment is an empty dream. Without fulfillment of legitimate desires, our disinterestedness leads only to uninterestedness, dispassion to depression, and self-surrender to self-pity. The West holds that however the East may brand the world as illusory and unreal, we know it to be all too real. That the saints and mystics struggle hard to overcome the lures and temptations of this world only shows that the world is real and has power. The human individual is not just a soul, but is body-mind-soul. For the West, liberation is cessation of suffering. As John Dewey said, when you are lost in the forest, the way out is the way by which you get out. Life calls for educating ourselves to face reality by knowing that we have nothing to rely on except our own power and potentiality. The West looks upon the Eastern way as life negating and depressive and its so-called moralism as weakness. Such a way engenders self-isolation, selfish individualism, and cowardly retreat from the challenges of life. The East is viewed as gloomy, fatalistic, impractical, and brooding.

The East responds by saying that the Western way, with its love of unrestrained pleasure, is suicidal. Its so-called life-asserting views only create speed without destination. In the name of reason, its philosophy goes in a circle. Its blind pragmatism seeks to nourish the body and mind at the cost of the soul. The greatness of a person is not to be judged by what that person does, but by what the person is. To the East, the West is viewed as shallow, drunk, noisy, and naive.

THE NEW VEDANTA COMBINING EAST AND WEST

Vivekananda saw the Western way as the missing counterpart of Vedanta. He admired the Western spirit—its penchant for heading into the future with courage and tenacity; its impatience—not waiting for things to happen but making them happen; and its readiness to take responsibility and risks, make mistakes, and forge ahead propelled by nothing but will. The swami loved America and the American spirit. He wrote:

> I love the Yankee land—I like to see new things. I do not care a fig to loaf about old ruins and mope a life out about old histories and keep sighing about the ancients. I have too much vigor in my blood for that. In America is the place, the people, the opportunity for everything new. I have become horribly radical.[7]

The pluck and thrust of the Western spirit fascinated Vivekananda. He passionately believed that the wisdom of the soul would never become a social reality without the support of the Western spirit, and that the Western way, unless guided toward the wisdom of the soul, would be the surest way to doom and destruction. Vedanta, in order to be complete, must combine the spirit of the East with that of the West. If the Vedic statement "All this is verily Brahman" is true, then the Vedic statement "That thou art" is equally true. Truth is to be realized through both knowledge and experience. Holiness and happiness are interrelated; meditation and action are complementary. Unselfishness is the greatest virtue and working for the good of others the highest form of worship. Self-mastery is the supreme austerity. Our direct experience of the Ultimate is our greatest savior, and the surest sign of direct experience is permanent transformation of character.

The most important contribution of the new Vedanta is its practicality. It replaces the humanitarian ideals of compassion and charity with the spiritual approach of service to the living God dwelling in the hearts of all beings. Practical Vedanta is a call to make the spiritual reality a social reality. Its essential teaching, in Swami Vivekananda's words, is as follows:

> Each soul is potentially divine. The goal is to manifest this divinity within by controlling nature: external and internal. Do this either by work, or worship, or psychic control, or philosophy—by one, or more, or all of these—and be free. This is the whole of religion. Doctrines, or dogmas, or rituals, or books, or temples, or forms, are but secondary details.[8]

The new Vedanta regards the four yogas—the paths of knowledge, devotion, selfless action, and concentration—as four independent paths leading to the goal of Self-knowledge, a departure from the old view that the first yoga is the highest and a culmination of the other three. The new approach not only declares that a human individual is divine but also has daring faith in that divinity. Practical Vedanta rejects the belief that the brain is an appendage of the genital gland, the view that leads to the neglect of the most important aspect of a human being: the soul. Practical Vedanta is not just a philosophy; it is a guideline for robust living, for being divine and also fully human. One cannot be divine without first being human.

The new Vedanta is available to all regardless of caste, color, creed, or race. Its practice does not require a person to have a male body and brahmin birth and to live in the seclusion of the forest. The old Vedanta says that one who does not believe in God is an atheist; the new Vedanta says, in the words of Swami Vivekananda, one who does not believe in oneself is an atheist. For the new Vedanta, material and spiritual development are conjoined. Work and worship go together. The inner and the outer dimensions of a person must be balanced in a pleasing harmony. The new approach does not believe in a God who promises a person eternal bliss in heaven but cannot give that person bread here. Practical Vedanta is an active spiritual quest—causing things to happen rather than letting them happen.

Swami Vivekananda foresaw that the East needed the West as much as the West needed the East—not only for success but also for survival. In his view, India possesses the wisdom of the soul but lacks a strong body to house that soul. The West, on the other hand, possesses a strong body but lacks soul. The soul and the body need to be united to make life meaningful. The West needs the wisdom of the soul so that its mighty achievements in science and technology will not prove self-destructive. The East needs Western muscle, vigor, vitality, human concern, and self-dignity for material regeneration. In the words of Swami Vivekananda, "By preaching the profound secrets of Vedanta in the Western world, we shall attract the sympathy and regard of these mighty nations, maintaining for ourselves the position of their teachers in spiritual matters; let them remain our teachers in all material concerns."[9]

Of the West, Swami Vivekananda wrote: "The present-day civilization of the West is multiplying day by day only the wants and distresses of men.... Nowhere have I heard so much of 'love, life, and liberty' as in this country [America], but nowhere is it less understood."[10] He predicted that within fifty years Europe would crumble to pieces if it did not mend its ways. Nearly fifty years after he had uttered this warning, the Second World War ended. Mere knowledge without understanding and love can lead to human catastrophe.

In his message to India, Swami Vivekananda called for strength: "Make your nerves strong. What we want is muscles of iron and nerves of steel. We have wept long enough. No more weeping, but stand on your feet and be men.... First of all, our young men must be strong. Religion will come afterwards. Be strong, my young friends; that is my advice to you. You will be nearer to heaven through football than through the study of the Gita."[11] Of Hinduism, he observed: "No religion on earth preaches the dignity of humanity in such a lofty strain as Hinduism, and no religion on earth treads upon the necks of the poor and low in such a fashion as Hinduism."[12]

THE NEW VEDANTA DRAWS FIRE

Vivekananda, with his new Vedanta, created a stir both in the East and in the West. While many universalists and scientifically minded persons in the West applauded his new message and the noble-minded breathed the air of spiritual freedom and spiritual democracy, the entrenched dogmatists denounced his teachings as monstrous and profane. They concocted false stories and spread rumors about his authenticity and personality and invented the "vilest of lies." It is said that "there was an attempt even to do away with him altogether by mixing poison with his coffee at a dinner in Detroit."[13] On his return to India, he recalled: "It struck me more than once that I should have to leave my bones on foreign shores, owing to the prevalence of religious intolerance."[14]

There were also attempts in India to suppress Vivekananda and his message. Leaders of orthodox Hindu society derided Vivekananda and his message of Vedanta as a veiled imitation of Christianity. They accused him of violations of caste rules and monastic traditions on the grounds that he had crossed the "black waters" of the ocean, lived in foreign lands, and dined with foreigners. His followers, the monks of the Ramakrishna Order—engaged in works of service nursing the sick, providing for the poor, and conducting epidemic and other relief work—were branded "scavenger monks," whose conduct was unworthy of the monastic life. Even some of the disciples of Sri Ramakrishna expressed doubt in the beginning about Vivekananda's new Vedanta, considering it a departure from their master's message. The followers of Vivekananda were but a handful of young men fired up by the spirit of worshipping the living God. They truly believed his message and were ready to die for their beliefs. Vivekananda's message prevailed: nothing could stop it because it answered the crying need of the time.

The same love that was born as Buddha, the Compassionate One, once again assumed a human form as Vivekananda. It was this unbounded love for suffering humankind that gave Vivekananda the mandate for his message. It gave him a power that nobody could match, a wisdom that no doctrine could qualify. Vivekananda's message bridged the gulf between the human being and God and broke through the wall that traditionally separates the physical from the spiritual. In him, the immortal message of the Upanishads and the Bhagavad Gita came to life again. Despair over degradation turned into hope for the future.

Truth must struggle hard against entrenched dogma, hardened superstitions, and credulous mass thinking. In spite of opposition, Vivekananda scattered the seeds of Vedanta wherever he went. Those seeds were not sown in vain. There are many societies and centers of Vedanta, both in the East and West, carrying the banner of the Ramakrishna Order. These centers are not merely houses of worship but homes of service where the living God is served with material, intellectual, and spiritual offerings.

In a prophetic mood, Vivekananda said that his message would sustain the world for the next fifteen hundred years. Science has shaken dogma-based religion to the very root. The decay of organized religion is in the air. In spite of all our technological achievements, there is a great spiritual void in the world today. The word *sermon* in the present-day Western world is an unpopular word, and a preacher is regarded by some as a salesperson. For many, the word *liberated* means liberated from all religions.

The myths and symbols that once gave emotional support to humankind have been shaken by the cold conclusions of science. After the Thirty Years' War, Europe lost faith in God, and after two world wars, humankind lost faith in itself. A culture of disbelief and skepticism has pervaded the world. Whatever claims the idealists put forth, the materialists try to disprove. No dogma-based religion can fill the spiritual void. What is needed is a spiritual teaching that can meet the challenges of science and secularism and make the spiritual quest meaningful for all. This is where the value of Vedanta lies.

Since the time of Vivekananda, Vedanta has silently but surely influenced the thought current of the world. When Vivekananda visited America, Robert Ingersoll, the famous orator and agnostic, told him: "Forty years ago you would have been hanged if you had come to preach in this country, or you would have been burnt alive. You would have been stoned out of the villages if you had come even much later."[15] But today the religions are engaged in continuous dialogue. At the present time, there is more consciousness of world unity than ever before. The voice of spirituality is becoming louder and louder, and the wave of spiritual democracy is breaking down the barrier of religiosity. Religious belief, for so long sure of its scriptural evidence, is now looking for the corroboration of science for its survival.

WORSHIP OF THE LIVING GOD

Vivekananda was the worshipper of the living God. He made God in the hearts of all the sole object of his worship. Even as a child, he would be overwhelmed to see the sufferings of the poor. To see and serve God in all became the passion of his youth, the dream of his wandering days. He lived with the poor masses of India, slept with them, ate with them, cried for their material salvation. Untiringly, he lobbied for them with his master, Sri Ramakrishna. Service of this living God was the joy of his last days. Like Prometheus, he brought down to earth the spiritual power from heaven for the benefit of all. This shifting of God from a far-off heaven to the human heart, as our innermost Self, marks a momentous advance in the spiritual history of the world.

Vivekananda passed away in 1902 before reaching the age of forty. But he left behind a promise for his living God:

And may I be born again and again, and suffer thousands of miseries, so that I may worship the only God that exists, the only God I believe in, the sum total of all souls. And above all, my God the wicked, my God the miserable, my God the poor of all races, of all species, is the especial object of my worship.[16]

It may be that I shall find it good to get outside my body—to cast it off like a worn-out garment. But I shall not cease to work. I shall inspire men everywhere, until the world shall know that it is one with God.[17]

4
Unity and Harmony of Religions

As part of the 1893 World's Fair Columbian Exposition held in the city of Chicago, a unique religious assembly was convened—the historic first World's Parliament of Religions. Never before in history had all the major religions of the world assembled to get to know one another, have a fruitful dialogue, and take a common stand for world unity and religious harmony. The 1893 parliament was organized as an afterthought of the Columbian Exposition planners and as a distant vision of ecumenism for some of the liberal-minded organizers, yet it became a dominant aspect of the exposition. The entire dynamic of the parliament changed because of the presence of one person—Swami Vivekananda, a visitor from the British colony of India. No one in recent history has so powerfully articulated and courageously defended religious harmony as has Swami Vivekananda. His message formed the keynote of the spiritual charter of East-West unity.

Swami Vivekananda came to the parliament as an independent individual to represent and defend the great teachers and prophets of all religions. Unknown, unattended, and without the support of any organization or religious denomination, he traveled to America. He slept in a boxcar, went unfed, and wandered through the streets of Chicago. Although he had no credentials from any religious body, he carried with him the message of his master, Sri

Ramakrishna, and a heart of cosmic proportion that could contain in it the whole universe. The unknown wanderer became famous overnight, following his appearance at the parliament. Newspapers, journals, and tabloids heralded his appearances and reported his words. To those present at the parliament and to the public at large, he became a champion of America's hopes and aspirations. People felt that before them stood one whom they had been seeking for years. The voice of Swami Vivekananda became the voice of the future. Before leaving India, Swami Vivekananda had indicated to some of his brother disciples and friends that the Parliament of Religions that was to take place in America was expressly for him. At that time, his words appeared to be only a wild dream or a fanciful vision. However, subsequent events proved the truth of the swami's words.

The theme of the parliament was the search for a durable basis for interfaith understanding and unity. What should be the nature of that unity? Can the religions of the world—so diverse in their beliefs and often so intolerant of one another—ever unite? Religious differences keep the world divided, inciting bitter hostility and hatred among people. While the prophets and saints proclaim the unity of the world and its people, their followers stubbornly uphold the differences. Religious intolerance unleashes diabolical hatred. Perversion of religious beliefs has impelled seemingly righteous people to come down to the level of brutes and commit acts of unimaginable cruelty. It has kindled the fires of religious wars, crusades, inquisitions, and ethnic cleansing. God has often been made to play the role of the commander of the army of the faithful, rather than that of loving Father and Mother of us all. It is often doubted whether the records of human history contain anything more horrible than the atrocities committed in the name of religion.

Religious conflict is driven by the narcissism of minor difference, in which essentially similar peoples exaggerate what separates them in a desperate search for identity. Religious harmony cannot easily compete with religious war fueled by hatred. Such war has an archetypal prestige. It has its bristling drama and exciting diction. Peace, however noble, has no glamour; its accoutrements are almost by definition unremarkable. The gospel of peace may be admired from a distance without its having much effect on daily behavior. The force that propels much of human action seems to be not love but hatred, brought about by the blood's need for vengeance.

Nonetheless, religious harmony has been the dream of all human beings. The world has tried to use economics, politics, and humanistic cooperation as a basis for unity, but these bonds of unity have not withstood the test of time. They have not survived the stresses of nationalistic and ethnic tensions. The nineteenth century witnessed the growth of political freedom, economic prosperity, and social reform, but also the decay of morality and spirituality. Against this backdrop of the helplessness of humanity, it is worth remembering Sri Ramakrishna's message of the harmony of all religions.

THE SEARCH FOR A COMMON GROUND

Three questions are often asked: Why are there so many religions? Why do they disagree? Is there any common ground where they can possibly meet?

In answer to the first question, different religions apparently evolved to suit the diversity of human temperaments, cultures, perspectives, and attitudes. Variety and plurality are the essence of our lives. The terrain of the human mind is extremely varied; no two minds are the same. Unity in diversity is the very law of nature, and the same law applies to religions. It would go against the dictates of reason and common sense to expect that all should think uniformly, or could be forced to do so. Thoughtful people generally differ, and difference of thought stimulates new thinking. Salvation or liberation, the promise of religion, is always individual because individually we are born, individually we experience pleasure and pain, and individually we die. So also, our approach to the Ultimate Reality is individual.

The second question is regarding the disagreements among religions. Religions differ greatly concerning their views of the Ultimate Reality, the meaning of creation, the way to salvation, and the nature of sacraments and ceremonies. Some look upon the Ultimate as a person having form, some as a personality with attributes but no form, some as formless Reality, some as void, and some as Pure Spirit. Regarding the meaning of creation, some insist upon the doctrine of absolute creation (God created the universe), some upon transformation of the Divine (a portion of God became the universe), and some upon illusory superimposition (creation is a projection of the individual mind on the Ultimate). Salvation for some is cessation of suffering, for others eternal life in heaven, and for still others it is the freedom of Self-knowledge attained in this very life. Some condemn rituals and ceremonies and some uphold them. Some view their faith as historical and regard that of others as merely mythological. Often it appears that the only thing religions have in common is their differences, and that the differences are irreconcilable.

The third question concerns the common ground where religions do meet. This common ground has four aspects: oneness of the Ultimate Reality, oneness of the goal, unanimity with regard to the divine nature of the soul, and the common virtues that are practiced by all.

All religions agree that the Ultimate Reality is one, whether it is looked upon as a person, void, or spirit, as having form or being formless. Those who believe that this Reality is God must agree that there is only one God, who is the God of all. It would be absurd to think that each faith has its own separate God. The different names and forms of God only represent frail human attempts to name the nameless and attribute forms and epithets to that which defies all forms and epithets.

The second aspect of the common ground is the oneness of the goal. The goal of all religion is God-consciousness, described variously as Self-knowledge, enlightenment, illumination, the beatific vision, union or communion with the Divine, and so forth. Spiritual progress is known by the increase of individual God-consciousness. Creeds, dogmas, sacraments, and rituals vary, but God-consciousness as the goal is common to all. This God-consciousness is more than theological or philosophical understanding or temporary emotion. True God-consciousness silences all doubt and transforms a person forever. Such a transformed person is called a free soul who wears no outward mark, and cannot be said to belong to any particular faith. Strictly speaking, we cannot designate Jesus as Christian, Buddha as Buddhist, or Sri Ramakrishna as Hindu. Just as at the center of a circle all the radii meet, so in God-consciousness all religions meet. The various accounts of God-consciousness are like photographs of the same building taken from different distances and different angles of vision. Each religion highlights a particular aspect of the Divine. No one religion can give finality to the nature of the Ultimate.

The third aspect of the common ground is the universal belief in the existence of a soul and its divinity. By following the disciplines of religion, we do not generate or acquire divinity, but gain faith in it. The spiritual quest is the manifestation of the divinity that is already in us. Virtue is that which helps us to manifest our divinity, and vice is that which blocks the manifestation.

The fourth aspect of the common ground is the fact that all religions, regardless of their doctrinal differences, exhort their followers to practice virtues such as love, compassion, purity, and holiness. Whether a person is a Hindu or a Christian, a Muslim or a Jew, a Buddhist or a Jain, a dualist or a non-dualist, these virtues remain the same.

The message of harmony emphasizes this common ground and considers the differences secondary details. It is based on the life, teaching, and spiritual experiences of Sri Ramakrishna. Sri Ramakrishna not only practiced the different paths of Hinduism, but also became the first spiritual sage in recorded history to follow the paths of other religions, such as Christianity and Islam, in faithful compliance with their respective creeds and disciplines. Following different religious paths, again and again Sri Ramakrishna reached the same goal, and so he declared: "As many faiths, so many paths."

According to Sri Ramakrishna, the spiritual goal is like the summit of a mountain, and the different religions are like different paths to reach that summit. This is harmony based on the common spiritual ground of all religions. All religions, to Sri Ramakrishna, are like different denominations of the one universal religion—the religion of God-consciousness. They belong to one and the same family and share an inviolable spiritual bond of harmony. This harmony is an eternal fact that only needs to be discovered. Differences with regard to views of the Ultimate and the meaning of creation are mere speculations of the human mind. They are details necessary in the early stages of spiritual growth. But as one begins to dive deep in search of truth, these details—myth, philosophy, rituals—lose their significance.

THE NATURE OF TRUE HARMONY

True religious harmony is different from eclectic harmony, which seeks to gather together only the non-conflicting elements of various faiths and bring them to a common denominator. Eclectic harmony is broad in its view, but is more intellectual than spiritual and practical. It ignores the diversity of culture and human disposition, and is not able to serve as a living religious teaching suitable for practice. At best, eclectic harmony is an anthology of religion. Another difficulty of eclectic harmony is that it becomes a sect of its own. The selected teachings of different religious systems that it tries to bring together eventually take the form of a new scripture. But such a collection of spiritual teachings cannot take the place of a religious scripture that derives its authority from the spiritual realization of a saint or a prophet. True harmony is never sectarian. Sectarian harmony is the harmony of uniformity. It suffers from narrowness of outlook, denies religious freedom, and advocates conversion of all to its belief. True harmony is not tolerance as a social necessity. One tolerates something or someone with reluctance, and therefore a meeting of minds is difficult or impossible.

True harmony is the harmony of principles rather than of personalities. It is a revelation rather than a formulation. True harmony does not deny the need for creed, philosophy, ritual, and dogma; it only asks the seeker to outgrow them. A tender plant needs fencing around, but the plant must outgrow the need for the fence. True harmony calls for acceptance and preservation of both unity and diversity, of both the summit of the mountain and the different pathways to it. True harmony is the realization of unity in the midst of diversity. It asks for recognition of the natural necessity of variation and for acceptance of the fact that truth can be expressed in a hundred different ways. It is harmony on the basis of the goal, leaving undisturbed the diversities of the paths to the goal.

True harmony is based on the spiritual oneness of existence. There is one life that pulsates in the whole universe. Spiritual oneness transcends the limitations of race, culture, creed, and dogma, and endows us with a unity that truly binds us. Again, true harmony is universal, applicable to all people of all time.

True harmony cannot be promoted merely by interfaith breakfasts or luncheons, by symposiums or conferences. These may stimulate the mind but do not alone achieve the goal. True harmony, in order to be a social reality, calls for deepening our individual spiritual consciousness. Religious dissension begins when the common goal, spiritual illumination, is forgotten or neglected. The further we move away from God, the greater will seem the differences between one religion and another; the nearer we move to God, the closer we shall feel to other religions. True harmony is not so much a fusion of religions as it is a fellowship of faiths based on the understanding and realization of the spiritual unity of the universe.

ROADBLOCKS TO INTERRELIGIOUS HARMONY

The root cause of interreligious dissension and hostility is dogmatism. Opposition to Jesus came not from another religion, but from the dogmatism of the Pharisees and Sadducees; Buddha's opponent was not Hinduism, but decadent Hindu dogmatism. Dogmatism has many faces and disguises: fanaticism that disclaims the rights of others, literalism that is rigid, liberalism that only skims the surface and explains away differences, and racial prejudice that claims cultural superiority.

There are fanatics who are eager to persecute those who do not share their particular brand of faith. Blinded by bigotry, they have tried to impose it upon others by propaganda, bribery, persuasion, force, or a combination of all these.

Then there are literalists who quarrel over doctrinal details and ignore the very goal of the religious quest. Anyone who disagrees with them is regarded as blasphemous; any doubter, however sincere and honest, is considered a fool, or worse, a heretic. Prompted by this narrow view, they brand others as heathens, untouchables, or pagans. Literalism easily degenerates into authoritarianism. It fails to see that truth is not opposed to reason and honest doubt, that knowledge of truth is incompatible with intolerance and hatred, and that salvation is the return to divinity and sobriety.

Liberalism that only skims the surface is another face of dogmatism. Such liberalism unconsciously takes its own point of view as the normative perspective for religion in general. It does not want to see that diversity and plurality are not mistakes and superstitions, and cannot be glossed over or explained away. Such liberals are often idealistic, and their idealism is at variance with the practical realities of the everyday world.

Racial and cultural prejudices are also enemies of interfaith understanding. Taken over by a sense of superiority, some races have thought that they alone represent true spirituality and that it was their mission to enlighten people of other races or cultures. Religious prejudice has often been fueled by such racial and cultural prejudice. It has made creed more important than deed, value more important than virtue.

Dogmatism in its various forms denounces the spirit of religious democracy and religious freedom. To convince others of its merit, dogmatism depends not upon logic and reason, but upon emotion and excitement. There is a saying that one who will not reason is a bigot, one who cannot is a fool, and one who dares not is a slave. Dogmatism is especially reprehensible with regard to that which is unknowable and indefinable. Dogmatism stands as an enemy common to all religions. True interfaith harmony calls for rising above dogmatism, returning to the original teachings of the prophets, and discovering the inherent spiritual unity of all religions. Interfaith dialogue in the spirit of true harmony is never a debate or an encounter, but a meeting of members of the same spiritual family—a grand reunion and a joyous celebration.

THE MESSAGE OF INTERFAITH HARMONY

Harmony of religions, once a dream of the noble-minded, has become the crying need of our time. Through improved means of communication, the world has become smaller and more pluralistic in every possible way. Cultural plurality and religious diversity without any enduring bond of spiritual unity are morally reprehensible, philosophically unjustifiable, and socially dangerous. The basis of this unity is spiritual oneness. Unless we develop morally and spiritually to the same degree that we have developed intellectually and technologically, our progress will only be toward disintegration and destruction.

Swami Vivekananda left us a legacy of unity and harmony. He called for a united stand against all forms of religious bigotry, intolerance, and dogmatism. His is the voice of truth, of the noblehearted men and women of all times, of the saints and prophets of all ages. As Swami Vivekananda declared at the Parliament of Religions:

> [I]f there is ever to be a universal religion, it must be one which will have no location in place or time; which will be infinite, like the God it will preach, and whose sun will shine upon the followers of Krishna and of Christ, on saints and sinners, alike; which will not be Brahminical or Buddhist, Christian or Mohammedan, but the sum total of all of these, and still have infinite space for development; which in its catholicity will embrace in its infinite arms, and find a place for every human being, from the lowest groveling savage, not far removed from the brute, to the highest man, towering by the virtues of his head and heart almost above humanity, making society stand in awe of him and doubt his human nature. It will be a religion which will have no place for persecution or intolerance in its polity, which will recognize divinity in every man and woman, and whose whole scope, whose whole force, will be centred in aiding humanity to realize its own true, divine nature.
>
> Offer such a religion and all the nations will follow you.... It was reserved for America to proclaim to all quarters of the globe that the Lord is in every religion.
>
> May He who is the Brahman of the Hindus, the Ahura-Mazda of the Zoroastrians, the Buddha of the Buddhists, the Jehovah of the Jews, the Father in heaven of the Christians, give strength to you to carry out your noble idea![1]

PART TWO

The Journey

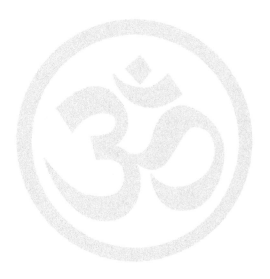

5
Love: Human and Divine

The spiritual quest has two aspects: theoretical and practical. The theoretical aspect is learning about the goal and deciding to make the journey. The practical aspect calls for total commitment to the spiritual goal and rigorous preparation for the journey to that goal. These preparations involve discriminating between the Real and the unreal, distinguishing love of God from self-love, taking care of our mind—our only companion on the journey—knowing our true friends along the path, observing the milestones of our progress, and being aware of the temptations and delusions that beset the journey. This journey is not possible unless a seeker is endowed with discrimination, renunciation, self-control, and sincere longing for the goal. Shankaracharya warns us about the dangers and difficulties along the path:

> The shark of hankering catches by the throat those seekers after liberation who have got only an apparent dispassion (*vairagya*) and are trying to cross the ocean of Samsara (relative existence), and violently snatching them away, drowns them half-way.[1]

> In the forest-tract of sense-pleasures there prowls a huge tiger called the mind. Let good people who have a longing for liberation never go there.[2]

Sri Ramakrishna reminds us of the one thing necessary to prepare for and proceed along the spiritual path: "Bhakti, love of God, is the essence of all spiritual discipline. Through love one acquires renunciation and discrimination naturally."[3]

LOVE: THE MOST POWERFUL CREATIVE FORCE

Love is the most powerful creative force in the universe. It is that force that connects a human individual with all. It is the power of love that overcomes all the negative forces of hatred, jealousy, and separateness, and binds everything and everybody into one unified whole. The language of love is unmistakable. Where there is love, there is no need of words. While the traders in religion speak of separateness and selfishness, the prophets and saints teach humanity the message of love. "As the Father hath loved me, so I have loved you; continue ye in my love.... This is my commandment, That ye love one another, as I have loved you" (John 15:9, 11). The power of love heals broken souls, broken homes, and mends the differences between people, societies, and cultures.

Through love, we seek union with others. The universe of living beings is like a huge tree. Individuals—whether subhuman, human, or superhuman—are like its leaves and branches. Their existence is one and indivisible. Through love we realize this organic connection of all in the universe, expand, and find fulfillment in life.

The urge for union with everything and everybody is irresistible. How we are to overcome separateness and aloneness has been the prime question of life for millennia. This question was the same for primitive human beings, nomadic human beings, peasants, traders, gamblers, and criminals. It was the same for medieval monks and nuns and ancient ascetics. Solutions have been sought through animal worship, military conquest, self-indulgence, ascetic renunciation, obsessive work, artistic creation, altruistic love, and love of God.

The feeling of separateness varies from person to person, and this variation is due to the degree of development of self-identity. To an infant, in whom I-consciousness is very little, the mother's physical presence is a solution. Persons who cannot think of anything beyond their physical existence identify with soil, plants, and nature. There are those who try to overcome this loneliness and separateness through drugs, trances, rituals, alcohol, and sex-gratification, but these are gross, violent, and fleeting, and their aftereffects are devastating. Still others try to overcome separateness by conformity with a group and the group's beliefs and practices. This is hiding in a herd—a form of union in which the individual disappears. Unity is not uniformity, which takes away the uniqueness of an individual and reduces everybody and everything to a standardized mass of human atoms, a form of suicide to overcome loneliness. Still others use activity as a form of union, as workers try to become united with the material they are working with. This unity, however, is not interpersonal and is therefore incomplete.

LOVE: THE BASIC URGE IN ALL LIVING BEINGS

Various ways to overcome separateness fail to reach their goal when the spiritual element of love is ignored or forgotten. The spiritual element is seeing the presence of the same soul or Self dwelling in all beings. Love, therefore, is the attraction of the part for the whole or the attraction of the whole for the part. In the *Brihadaranyaka Upanishad,* the great sage Yajnavalkya tells his wife:

> Verily, not for the sake of the husband, my dear, is the husband loved, but he is loved for the sake of the self [which, in its true nature, is one with the Supreme Self]. Verily, not for the sake of the wife, my dear, is the wife loved, but she is loved for the sake of the self.[4]

The Bible says, "Thou shalt love thy neighbor as thyself" (Matt. 19:19). The meaning is that the same Self dwells in both you and your neighbor. Our sense of purity and impurity depends upon the depth of this Self-knowledge.

The natural urge of love is cosmocentric, which means loving all with same-sightedness without distinction. But because of the lack of knowledge of the spiritual element, the free flow of love becomes tainted, perverted, and degraded to selfish, human love. Such love becomes egocentric. The emotions and urges of anger, lust, jealousy, and hatred are negative reactions, and the root cause of all of them is egocentric love. Hell is often described as a place where the creatures fail to love one another.

FORMS OF SELFISH HUMAN LOVE

Human love, when tainted by selfish motives and desires, can take many familiar forms:

Selfish love is *self-love* that distorts one's view of oneself. Such self-love becomes possessive when the object of love is viewed as property and used for the lover's self-interest. Possessive love is guided by deep attachment and delusion. Parents can love their children as their property. In some societies, parents love their son more than their daughter solely because he is expected to support them in their old age and difficult times. If the son prematurely becomes disabled or struck with a mortal illness, the love of the parents begins to diminish. Parents often try to fulfill through their children the desires that they themselves could not fulfill.

Idolatrous love manifests itself when a person makes of the loved one a hero or an idol. When, however, reality fails to meet the idealized expectations, the object of love is discarded and a new idol is sought.

Receptive love is a third form of selfish human love. In receptive love, a person wants to receive but not give love, wants to be loved but does not think of being lovable. Receptive love is devoted but dependent, obedient but parasitic.

A fourth form of self-love is *sentimental love*. Sentimental love lacks the very basis of love. It is fleeting, unsteady, and careless. It has no root and no depth. Such love is guided by emotional attachment; the lover expects the object of love to share his or her every emotion. When this does not occur, sentimental love deteriorates into hatred.

Finally, there is *idealistic love.* Idealistic love is immature and unrealistic and does not want to acknowledge imperfections. No human individual is perfect. You cannot love a person unless you love the person as a whole and accept the person's imperfections as part of his or her personality. When idealistic love realizes the imperfections of the loved person, he or she becomes disillusioned.

MARKS OF TRUE LOVE

True love has its own marks. It is unity in diversity. In true love, the two become one, yet remain two. True love is active; but mere activity without motivation does not tell the whole story. It is giving, not receiving. The noted psychoanalyst Erich Fromm aptly describes the marks of true love as care, responsibility, respect, and knowledge:

> That love implies *care* is most evident in a mother's love for her child. No assurance of her love would strike us as sincere if we saw her lacking in care for the infant ... and we are impressed by her love if we see her caring for the child.... *Love is the active concern for the life and the growth of that which we love....*

> Care and concern imply another aspect of love; that of *responsibility.* Today responsibility is often meant to denote duty.... But responsibility, in its true sense, is an entirely voluntary act; it is my response to the needs, expressed or unexpressed, of another human being. To be "responsible" means to be able and ready to "respond." ... He feels responsible for his fellow men, as he feels responsible for himself....

Responsibility could easily deteriorate into domination and possessiveness, were it not for a third component of love, *respect*. Respect is not fear and awe; it denotes, in accordance with the root of the word (*respicere* = to look at), the ability to see a person as he is....

To respect a person is not possible without *knowing* him; care and responsibility would be blind if they were not guided by knowledge. Knowledge would be empty if it were not motivated by concern.... It is possible only when I can transcend the concern for myself and see the other person in his own terms.[5]

True love is loving everyone equally. It is seeing the presence of the *Ishta* (worshipped form of God) or the Atman (one's own true Self) in all.

Sri Ramakrishna makes a distinction between self-love and divine love with the words *maya* and *daya*. Maya is love for others driven by attachment and possessiveness. *Daya* is compassion. It is love for others without any selfish motivation or expectation:

There is a great difference between daya, compassion, and maya, attachment. Daya is good, but not maya. Maya is love for one's relatives—one's wife, children, brother, sister, nephew, father, and mother. But daya is the same love for all created beings without any distinction.[6]

Loving others requires the capacity to identify ourselves with others. This again depends upon being one's own Self. Liberation is essentially the liberation of love from the drags of self-love.

As marks of true love, Swami Vivekananda describes:

We may represent love as a triangle, each of the angles of which corresponds to one of its inseparable characteristics. There can be no triangle without its three angles, and there can be no true love without its three following characteristics. The first angle of our triangle of love is that love knows no bargaining. Wherever there is any seeking for something in return, there cannot be any real love; it becomes a mere matter of shopkeeping....

The second angle of the triangle of love is that love knows no fear. Those who love God through fear are the lowest of devotees—not fully developed men....

The third angle of the triangle of love is that love knows no rival, for in it is always embodied the lover's highest ideal.[7]

Life stories of the prophets and saints give us epic examples of true love. The following are some of these examples.

The love of Christ for his disciples

Christ showered true love upon his disciples. Before his crucifixion, he prophesied that all of his disciples would desert him, one of them would betray him to the Romans for thirty pieces of silver, and some would deny him. Those who have read the Bible know that all Christ's prophecies came to be true. He died a lonely death on the cross. Yet his love for his disciples remained the same. He promised them that he would be with them until the end of time. "Teaching them to observe all things whatsoever I have commanded you: and, lo, I am with you always, even unto the end of the world" (Matt. 28:20).

Saint Durgacharan's love for his master Sri Ramakrishna

Durgacharan Nag was a humble devotee and disciple of Sri Ramakrishna. Sri Ramakrishna described him as a flaming fire of devotion. Whenever he would come to see Sri Ramakrishna, he would be overwhelmed with spiritual emotion, his body would tremble, and he would be unable to speak. He saw Sri Ramakrishna as the divine Lord in human form. Readers of *The Gospel of Sri Ramakrishna* may recall Sri Ramakrishna's prophecy before his death. Sri Ramakrishna was dying with cancer of the throat. Out of love, he gave those who came to him much more than they deserved. M. describes Sri Ramakrishna's suffering as another crucifixion—a sacrifice of the body for the sake of the devotees.

Sri Ramakrishna looks at the devotees and his love for them wells up in a thousand streams. Like a mother showing her tenderness to her children, he touches the face and chin of Rakhal and Narendra.

A few minutes later he says to M., "If the body were to be preserved for a few days more, many people would have their spirituality awakened."

He pauses a few minutes.

"But this is not to be. This time the body will not be preserved."

The devotees eagerly await the Master's next words.

"Such is not the will of God. This time the body will not be preserved, lest, finding me guileless and foolish, people should take advantage of me, and lest I, guileless and foolish as I am, should give away everything to everybody. In this Kaliyuga, you see, people are averse to meditation and japa."[8]

During the Master's stay at Cossipore, Nag Mahasay [Saint Durgacharan Nag] saw him a few times. His visits were not frequent, for he could not bear to see the unspeakable sufferings of the Master. One day Sri Ramakrishna saw him entering the room and said, "Come near. Sit close to me." He warmly embraced Nag Mahasay for some minutes. Another day finding him at his bedside, the Master said, "Look here, Durgacharan. The doctors have failed. Can you do anything to cure me?" Nag Mahasay reflected for a minute and then resolved to transfer the Master's disease into his own body. He said in an animated voice, "Yes, sir, I know how to cure you. By your grace I will do it at once." And he approached the Master. Sri Ramakrishna divined his purpose and pushed him back saying, "Yes, I know you can do that."[9]

After Sri Ramakrishna passed away, Durgacharan stopped eating. He remained lying down, covering himself with a blanket. Narendra and the other disciples came to his residence and fervently requested him to eat. At this, Durgacharan took one of his earthen cooking pots and hit himself on the head. Bitterly crying, he said, "What good is there by giving food to this body that will see the Master no more?"

Holy Mother's transforming power of love

Swami Nikhilananda, one of Holy Mother's (Sri Sarada Devi's) direct disciples, narrates the following incident about Mother's love for a devotee:

[A] Moslem, Amjad, who was a bandit, built the wall for Holy Mother's new house. One day she invited him for a meal, which was arranged on the porch of her house. An orthodox Hindu in many respects treats a Moslem as untouchable and regards food or drink touched by him as polluted. Nalini, Holy Mother's niece, began to throw the food at Amjad's plate from a distance. Holy Mother noticed this and said: "How can one enjoy food if it is offered with such scorn? Let me wait on him properly." After he had finished his meal, Holy Mother cleaned the place with her own hands. Nalini shrieked: "Aunt, you have lost your caste!" "Keep quiet," the Mother scolded her. And she added: "As Sarat is my son, exactly so is Amjad." Sarat was a direct disciple of Sri Ramakrishna, the Secretary of the Ramakrishna Mission, and a monk possessed of saintly virtues, and Amjad was a man of disreputable character. Her behaviour on this occasion bears out her remark: "I am the Mother of the good and I am the Mother of the wicked."[10]

Swami Vivekananda's love for Sri Ramakrishna

Swami Saradananda, a direct disciple of Sri Ramakrishna, describes the following example of Swami Vivekananda's love for his Master.

The Master ... used to busy himself about Narendra [Swami Vivekananda] when the latter came to Dakshineswar. The moment he saw Narendra at a distance his entire mind would run out of his body, as it were, with great speed and bound him with an embrace of love. It is impossible to say on how many occasions we saw the Master go into samadhi saying, "There's Na—, there's Na—." Still, there came a time, even before very close intimacy developed, when Narendra would come to the Master, but the latter was supremely indifferent to him. Narendra came, bowed down to the Master, sat in front of him and waited long. The Master looked at him but once and sat wholly indifferent, without even inquiring about his welfare, let alone expressing his loving concern for him. Narendra thought that the Master was perhaps under the influence of spiritual emotions. Having waited long, he came out of the room and began talking with Sri Hazra and smoking. Hearing that the Master was talking with others, Narendra came back to him. But the Master did not speak a word to him and lay down on his bed with his face turned in the opposite direction! The whole day passed that way and evening approached, still Narendra found no change in the Master's attitude. So, he bowed down to him and returned to Calcutta.

Hardly had a week elapsed when Narendra came again to Dakshineswar to find the Master in the same mood. On that occasion also he spent the whole day in various talks with Hazra and others, and started home before dusk. Narendra came for the third and fourth time, without finding the slightest change in the attitude of the Master. But, without feeling at all distressed or wounded on account of it, he continued paying visits to the Master as usual. The Master sent from time to time some one to bring the news of Narendra's welfare when the latter was staying at home, but he continued to behave towards him in that manner for some time more, whenever he would come to him. At the end of more than a month when the Master saw that Narendra did not desist from visiting Dakshineswar, he had him called to him one day and asked, "Well, I do not speak even a single word to you; still you come. Why so?" Narendra said, "Do I come here to hear you speak? I love you; I wish to see you; that is why I come." Highly pleased with the reply, the Master said, "I was testing you to see whether you would cease coming if you did not get the proper love and attention. It is only a spiritual aspirant of your order who can put up with so much (neglect and indifference). Any one else would have left me long ago and would have never come here."[11]

TRANSFORMATION OF HUMAN LOVE TO DIVINE LOVE

Human love reaches its highest fulfillment when the loved one is looked upon as the human face of the Divine. The divine Self dwells in the heart of all living beings, and this Self is adored and worshipped by different names, such as Pure Consciousness, God, Pure Spirit, and Purusha.

Vedanta describes the universe as *Virat,* the cosmic body of the Divine. God is the sum total of all souls, and different souls are sparks of that Supreme Soul. They are eternally connected to the Supreme. The Upanishads describe the Supreme Soul: "His hands and feet are everywhere; His eyes, heads, and faces are everywhere; His ears are everywhere; He exists compassing all."[12] Knowers of truth feel as if they walk through a million feet, eat through a million mouths, and hear through a million ears, being united with all beings and things of the universe.

When a person achieves this realization, he or she then transfers all attachment and attention to this divine Self and the love for the beings and things of this universe flows through the Supreme Self. But this transference is preceded by an awakening that lets a person see and know that no one in this relative universe really loves us or can love us truly. As Sri

Ramakrishna says, "When a man is seized with the spirit of intense renunciation, he regards the world as a deep well and his relatives as venomous cobras."[13] Swami Vivekananda in his poem "To a Friend" describes the transformation of human love to divine love:

O selfless lover, great of heart,
Know thou, within this sordid world
There is no room at all for thee:
Could a frail marble bust endure
The blow an anvil's mass will bear?
Be as one slothful, mean, and vile,
With honeyed tongue but poisoned heart,
Empty of truth and self-enslaved—
Then thou wilt find thy place on earth....

From highest Brahman to the worm,
Even to the atom's inmost core,
All things with Love are interfused.
Friend, offer body, mind, and soul
In constant service at their feet.
Thy God is here before thee now,
Revealed in all these myriad forms:
Rejecting them, where seekest thou
His presence? He who freely shares
His love with every living thing
Proffers true service unto God.[14]

Shankaracharya says in his "Hymn of Renunciation":

While man supports his family,
See what loving care they show!
But when his aging body falters,
Nearing the time of dissolution,
None, not even his nearest kin,
Will think to ask him how he fares.

Worship Govinda,* worship Govinda,
Worship Govinda, foolish one![15]

The awakening described above makes a person direct all love to the divine Self, by whose will we are born, who nurtures and sustains us while we are alive, who is the goal of all our desires and aspirations, and who, wearing many disguises, surrounds us in this world. This revelation prompts a person to practice the spiritual disciplines of nonattachment and selflessness in order to free himself or herself from the bondage of selfish and ego-centric love.

The spiritual quest is essentially a quest for the liberation of our love. By loving all beings and things as the divine Self, a mortal becomes immortal. His or her life becomes blessed. The world no longer appears as a framework of delusion but as the true kingdom of God.

---

*An epithet of Sri Krishna.

6

The Human Mind and Its Health

To proceed on the spiritual journey, we need to develop physical, mental, and spiritual strength. We are constantly reminded of the need for physical health and fitness. Hundreds of publications caution us about the consequences of not maintaining physical fitness. They offer us health foods, dietary supplements, and advise us to exercise every day. We keep busy selecting the proper nutrition in order to keep our bodies fit; some of us exercise regularly in order to maintain our physical fitness. We are very aware of the fact that good health is the greatest insurance against disease, disability, and other problems that may affect our physical body. But rarely do we think of our mental health and fitness, which serve as the greatest insurance against the harsh realities of life: anxiety, fear, uncertainty, illness, old age, and death. We forget that when we neglect the mind, it invariably becomes weak and out of control, making us unfit in every aspect of our lives. A weak mind runs the risk of aging prematurely.

The Bhagavad Gita reminds us of the importance of the mind and its control:

Let a man be lifted up by his own self; let him not lower himself; for he himself is his friend, and he himself is his enemy.

To him who has conquered himself by himself, his own self is a friend, but to him who has not conquered himself, his own self is hostile, like an external enemy.[1]

The Yoga system describes five types of mind: dull, scattered, excited, concentrated, and suspended. A dull mind is overpowered by inertia. The scattered mind is out of control. The excited mind is constantly agitated by its passions and delusions. But the concentrated mind is sharp and one-pointed, and the suspended mind gravitates toward absorption. The first three types are unsuitable in both worldly and spiritual matters. Only the last two are fit for spiritual pursuit. The healthy and fit mind has ten fundamental aspects:

• Ability to adjust to changing situations and circumstances

• Capacity to concentrate and detach at will

• Control over raw emotions, urges, and impulses

• Keenness of perception and sharpness of memory

• Forbearance and frustration-bearing capacity

• Ability to overcome loneliness and emotional dependence

• Mature ego that is free from infantile self-incrimination and adolescent self-aggrandizement

• Freedom from the herd complex that prevents a person from developing self-identity

• High degree of efficiency in performance

• Innovative spirit and capacity to learn from others

Animals depend upon physical strength. Saints and prophets possess soul strength. But human beings are heavily dependent on their strength of mind, and strength of mind depends upon its health.

When the physical body becomes weak, it becomes susceptible to disease and decay; when the mind becomes weak, it becomes prey to a host of problems, such as depression and lack of self-control. A weak mind acts against our peace, happiness, and well-being. By allowing our mind to become weak, we contribute fifty percent to our problems, and the external world contributes fifty percent. We have no control over the external world, but we can strengthen our minds and thus maintain control of our fifty percent.[2]

GUIDELINES FOR THE HEALTH OF THE MIND

Barring pathological or genetic deficiencies, the health of the body and mind depend upon the five factors of diet, exercise, conservation, rest, and moderation.

Diet

Give the mind balanced nutrition. Like the body, the mind must be fed with a healthy, nutritious diet. The mind draws its nutrition through the five organs of perception—the organs of sight, sound, touch, taste, and smell—and this nutrition must be healthy. A mental diet that helps the mind exert control over the body is considered healthy. The mind must receive this healthy diet on a daily basis.

In daily life, an average person cannot avoid worldly company and conversation. Remaining in the world of delusion and desire, the mind unconsciously absorbs worldly propensities. To counteract this mental absorption, a person must seek holy company, hear holy conversation, and practice meditation on the Self daily—all in order to cleanse the mind by pouring holy thoughts into it.

The Bhagavad Gita uses three terms to outline the items of diet that affect our body and mind: *sattva* (tranquility), *rajas* (restlessness), and *tamas* (inertia). A *sattvika* diet is healthy because it promotes vitality of the body and peace of mind; a *rajasika* diet, however, creates passion; and a *tamasika* diet, lethargy.

Diet for the mind must be *sattvika*. Both material and mental food that heighten soul awareness instead of body awareness are regarded as *sattvika* and healthy. The *Uddhava Gita* speaks of ten factors that help increase the *sattva* quality of the mind:

> Scripture, water, people, place, time, work, birth [i.e., spiritual rebirth], meditation, mantra, and purification—these are the ten causes which develop the gunas....

> For the increase of *sattva* a man should concern himself with *sattvika* things alone. Thence comes spirituality, and from this again knowledge—pending the realisation of one's independence and the removal of the superimposition of gross and subtle bodies.[3]

Sattvika scriptures are those that teach renunciation of desires and oneness with the Ultimate Reality; *sattvika* water is holy water, not liquor or wine; *sattvika* people are spiritual people, not the worldly minded or wicked; a *sattvika* place is solitary and peaceful; *sattvika* time is in the early morning, early evening, or any such time available for the practice of meditation; *sattvika* work is unselfish work, not work for one's own interest; *sattvika* birth is initiation into pure and noninjurious forms of religion whose goal is God-realization—and nothing else; *sattvika* meditation is only on the Lord, not on sense objects; a *sattvika* mantra, or sacred word, is Om; and *sattvika* purification is purification not just of the body but, most importantly, of the mind.

Exercise

Exercise your mind to prevent mental aging. When we do not exercise our muscles, they get flabby. In the same way, when we do not stimulate our minds with new challenges, we lose fitness for optimal function.

Exercise control over the instincts of palate and sex. The mind loses its vigor by giving in to these urges. By refusing to be bullied by these urges and by withstanding their impacts, the mind develops its moral muscles. As the Bhagavad Gita says: "He who is able to withstand the force of lust and anger even here before he quits the body—he is a yogi, he is a happy man."[4]

Learn to adjust and maintain flexibility of mind. In our personal and social lives, things do not always happen according to our liking. We must learn to accept changes without sacrificing our basic principles. Flexibility is the sign of a youthful mind. When persons grow mentally old, they become rigid and lose flexibility. In family life, they expect everyone to adjust to them. In the workplace, they expect their colleagues to cater to their old-fashioned thoughts, ideas, and whims. Since these expectations can never be fulfilled, such persons often become hypercritical and unhappy.

Practice patience under all circumstances. Act and do not react. Patience is a sign of strength. Weak-minded persons become easily angered, influenced by passions, and intolerant of others. Out of impatience, they often say or do something that they later regret. The practice of patience helps to develop strength of mind.

Exercise control over your emotions. Emotions control us too much. Strength of mind is measured in terms of control over our emotions, both good and bad. Weak-minded persons become victims of the upsurges and down-surges of their emotions because of their weak nerves. Such persons may feel great spiritual emotion by hearing a devotional song or spiritual discourse and may shed tears and feel a spiritual thrill. But the same persons are susceptible to the down-surges of their minds and may fall victim to feelings of lust, greed, anger, and jealousy.

Develop self-identity. Weak-minded persons have no self-identity and therefore no individuality. Such persons try to shine in the borrowed light of others by imitating others. They follow the unthinking masses. The growth of personality is the growth of the mind, and the growth of the mind is measured by the ability to give up the herd instinct and think independently.

Be in the company of those who are mentally brighter, stronger, and have higher flights of mind. A usual sign of a person's mental decline is a preference to be in the company of those with lower flights of mind. The development of mental muscles requires facing obstacles and overcoming them. The secret of success is to learn to accept the impossible and bear with the intolerable.

Be creative and innovative. A healthy mind is creative, innovative, and eager to find alternate ways to solve a problem. Such a mind has the capacity to meet problems without being dismayed, patiently endure pain and suffering, and face unfavorable circumstances without floundering. With the decline of mental capacity, an individual loses these qualities and becomes prone to follow the beaten track. A fatigued mind has no choice but to repeat and copy.

Maintain the capacity of the mind. Persons of average intelligence should finish a simple project within a reasonable length of time. But with mental decline, they will need more and more time to complete a project they would have done in much less time some years earlier. In order to maintain the capacity of the mind, persons are called upon to perform actions with speed yet with efficiency and quality.

Keep yourself occupied. An idle mind lapses into inertia, daydreaming, and fanciful imaginations. The best occupation is spiritual; the next best is intellectual or selfless activity. For this reason, beginners on the spiritual quest must not have a huge block of unused time to deal with. What is important in prayer and meditation is conscious concentration. Seekers should be fully aware of their mind's activities. It is easier for beginners to spend a shorter, more concentrated amount of time in spiritual practice.

Be a good performer. The Bhagavad Gita describes yoga as efficiency in performance. A yogi is integrated, temperate, and efficient. Athletes cannot afford to play poorly because fans in the stadium are not cheering them on. Physicians cannot afford to be inattentive because they are not receiving a large fee. Good performers will always perform well, irrespective of the situation. An action is considered good if performed with naturalness, efficiency, and grace.

Never lose the spirit of learning. Sri Ramakrishna said, "As long as I live, so long do I learn."[5] The ability to learn from others is a characteristic mark of a healthy mind. It is a sign of life and growth. When we begin to think that we know best, we show an unmistakable sign of mental deterioration.

Forbear, forbear, forbear. Bear with frustration, criticism, loneliness, and despair. A person's frustration-bearing capacity is a sign of mental strength. So is the capacity to bear with criticism. It is said that friends make us glad, but critics make us think.

Overcome loneliness. A healthy mind is guided by a mature ego that is relatively free from various dependencies, whereas infantile or adolescent egos are highly dependent and dominating. Such egos cannot bear being alone. They must be entertained, flattered, and praised, or else they feel miserable.

Develop mental insurance against the harsh realities of life. Yoga and Vedanta advise us to have an insurance policy against the maladies of the mind. This insurance cannot be bought from any outside agency by paying a premium; such insurance has to be developed within by keeping contact with our true Self through the practice of Self-awareness, backed up by the practices of nonattachment and self-control. That we will have to face the harsh realities of life is inevitable and universal, a natural law of the material world, and must be accepted with equanimity. Fear of old age is to be overcome by realizing that we are not our egoself but our true, ageless Self or soul. Fear of death is to be overcome by meditating on this immortal, all-pervading Self. In meditation, we learn to die both physically and mentally, in a measured way, by our detachment from our body and mind. With each contact we make with our true Self, we create a memory of it in our mind, and these memories are the greatest mental insurance against uncertainty, sorrow, pain, old age, and death.

Only a naïve or ignorant person expects everything in life to be smooth and favorable. A mature person knows that sorrow and joy, pain and pleasure, life and death, and other pairs of opposites are the unalterable laws of life, and such a person prepares for them through the practice of *tapasya,* or austerity. Physical austerity is bearing all the physical suffering and pain we know to be universal and a part of life. Mental austerity is maintaining evenness of mind in the face of adverse circumstances and withstanding the impacts of gross urges without being overcome by them. By bearing with the intensities of these gross urges, we develop our mental and moral muscles.

Conservation

Conservation of mental energy calls for the practice of self-mastery. It is asserting our soul strength over raw impulses. The time that we devote to *japa,* meditation, and selfless service purifies our physical energy and converts it into mental energy, and mental energy into spiritual energy. This purified spiritual energy that remains stored in the brain is called *ojas. Ojas* endows a person with great power and vitality of mind. The more the energy is purified, the easier it is to conserve.

Rest

The body needs rest for recuperation from wear and tear. Nature daily forces us to go to sleep so that we can wake up with fresh energy. The same law applies to the mind. The mind should detach itself from the sense organs and become attached to the Self for its rest. When we practice detachment in meditation, we want to relax consciously. Withdrawal and response are the two movements of our mind. A weak mind loses the capacity to detach and, therefore, also loses the capacity to attach. The detached mind, being in communion with its true Self, recharges itself with new vigor and is never overwhelmed by the changes of life.

Moderation

We are often prone to act in an extreme way; therefore, moderation is to be exercised in all matters. Mental habits do not change overnight. Character is not formed in a single day. Our mind must cooperate with us in our endeavor. Austerities and spiritual disciplines, when practiced too little, do not produce any effect on the body and mind. On the other hand, when practiced in an extreme way, they can provoke reactions from the body and mind. Hence, moderation is vital in caring for the mind. Steady, regulated, and persistent care can help the mind to regain its moral and spiritual strength.

According to Yoga and Vedanta, the mind is our second body and care of its health and fitness is necessary if it is to accompany us on the spiritual journey toward the goal of Self-knowledge. Lack of care for the mind makes the mind weak, and weakness of the mind is the sole cause of our miseries and sufferings in life. In the Bhagavad Gita, Arjuna tells Sri Krishna, "the mind, O Krishna, is restless, turbulent, powerful, and obstinate. To control it is as hard, it seems to me, as to control the wind." But Sri Krishna assures us, "Doubtless, O mighty Arjuna, the mind is restless and hard to control; but by practice and by detachment ... it can be restrained."[6]

7
Human Relations:
A Spiritual Guide

In chapter 5, we discussed the nature of true love, human and divine. Now we turn our attention to the proper health of a spiritual seeker's relationships with others.

Human beings are created to live together in peace and harmony, and our behavior plays a vital role in that regard. Behavior makes a difference in human relations, social exchanges, company, conversation, family atmosphere, workplace atmosphere, and all conceivable circumstances. Our behavior in a given situation expresses our thoughts and feelings and includes our actions and reactions. Through our behavior we can make enemies of friends or friends of enemies, connect with others or isolate ourselves from everybody and everything.

Right behavior is an expression of our character, upbringing, and culture. It is not artificial politeness, pretentious dignity, or diplomatic kindness. Right behavior is marked by integrity, honesty, humility, and straightforwardness. These are the natural qualities of a person of good character. A good person will be good at all times and in all situations. It is true that codes of civility in behavior vary from one society to another and also within the same society. What is well known to a native may puzzle a foreigner. The offering of the hand by a person, which was originally intended to show that he or she carried no weapon, and the uncovering of the head, which originally showed defense-lessness, are considered good manners in one society but meaningless in another. Yet all civil manners and behavior have one common goal—respect for and recognition of others. The language and symbols may vary, but the norms of morality remain the same.

Right behavior is a social necessity. It preserves the spirit of cooperation without which there would be a disintegration of social values and stability. A human individual is born not into a bare physical universe but into a world of human values, human purposes, human instruments, and human design. All that we know or believe about the physical world is a result of our own personal and social development. The path of personal development has been from selfishness to selflessness, from herd-like cohesion to rational cooperation, and from inhibition to freedom.

Right behavior is a psychological necessity. A person cannot be happy being isolated from others. It is not how much a person knows but how that person behaves that is of the utmost importance. Despite talent and brilliance, a person can become a failure because of indecent behavior.

Right behavior is a spiritual necessity. It is vital for realizing our true Self in love and respect for others. Vedanta teaches us that the basis of all ethics is seeing the reflection of one's own Self in all. Sri Krishna says in the Bhagavad Gita, "Him I hold to be the supreme yogi, O Arjuna, who looks on the pleasure and pain of all beings as he looks on them in himself."[1] Self-realization is the one goal of life. Practice of righteous conduct, cultivation of moral values, fulfillment of legitimate desires, and achievement of worldly success—all find their consummation in the realization of our true Self. Through Self-realization, we find our connection with the cosmos. The path to Self-realization is a graded one. One is first required to be a good person, then an ethical person, then a moral person, and finally a spiritual person. One who does not care for one's fellow human beings will not care for God.

DETERMINANTS OF BEHAVIOR

Behavior is a reflection of the character of a person, but the question remains as to what determines character. There are differences of views in this regard.

One view says that character is determined by the mind of a person, and the mind functions according to temperament and endocrine secretions. The mind, according to this view, is a by-product of the brain. It is born with the body and also dies with the body. The chemical and glandular secretions depend upon a person's heredity, culture, and upbringing. This view denies the existence of the soul or any form of psyche beyond the body.

A second view says character is an extension of the mind. The mind, according to this view, is born with the body like a clean slate without any past impressions. Heredity, environment, education, and upbringing help in the full formation of the mind. But this view does not explain the inequalities that persist in different individuals born in the same family and raised in the same environment with a similar education and upbringing. No doubt heredity and environment influence the mind heavily. But to say that these are the constituent elements of the mind would be unrealistic.

A third view says character is the expression of the mind, and the mind acts and reacts in a given situation, driven by its urges. Generally speaking, the urges are five: self-preservation, self-expression, sex gratification, gregariousness, and knowledge. Among these urges, there is a master urge. The master urge, according to some, is the instinct of sex, to others, the desire for pleasure, and to still others, the drive for power. This view asserts that our conscious mind acts and reacts influenced by the subconscious and its urges. This view also denies the spiritual element in a person's character: the soul and its urge to expand for self-fulfillment.

In contrast to these views, Yoga and Vedanta maintain the following:

- The mind of a person is different from the body.

- Each person is born with a blueprint of mind, carried from previous lives.

- The mind is comprised of memories and *samskaras,* or subtle tendencies, that create urges and reactions in the mind in a given situation.

- A human individual is essentially soul or Self, which uses the body and mind as the instruments for self-expression and self-fulfillment.

- The mind, like the body, is material in structure and has no consciousness of its own. It acts and reacts using the borrowed power of the Self, which is the only conscious element in a person.

- There are three levels of the mind: subconscious, conscious, and superconscious. Rising above the subconscious and conscious states, a person reaches the superconscious, wherefrom he or she perceives reality in its pristine purity.

- The master urge in a person is neither sex gratification nor pleasure nor power but Self-realization, which guarantees the supreme fulfillment of life, maximum enjoyment, eternal life, unalloyed pleasure, and knowledge.

- The mind, being material, is subject to the law of the *gunas,* known as *sattva* (tranquility), *rajas* (activity), and *tamas* (inertia).

YOGA AND VEDANTA AND HUMAN CHARACTER

Yoga and Vedanta teach us that our character is known by the different proportions and combinations of the three *gunas,* which are constantly changing due to our way of living. The three *gunas* have been compared to three strands of a rope that bind the soul to the world. To a certain degree, all three *gunas* are present in the mind, and they are the cause of our delusion, attachment, and suffering. *Tamas* is like a veil that altogether blocks our perception of Reality and is the greatest cause of ignorance and indolence. *Rajas* rises by overcoming *tamas* but creates many fantasies, desires, ambitions, and delusions. *Sattva* manifests itself by overcoming *tamas* and *rajas*. When *sattva* prevails, a person gets a clear perception of reality, and is driven toward realizing the nature of the Self. In this regard, human personalities fall under three broad categories, according to their respective *guna* composition.

Tamasika (dull and dark) persons are generally withdrawn, introverted, pessimistic, and passive. They have an inherent inferiority complex, a lack of self-confidence, infantile demands, and are heavily narcissistic. By nature, they are melancholy and self-incriminating. They dwell on the troubles and dangers of life and ignore its bright side. They are quickly discouraged by setbacks and unpleasant experiences and are easily put to flight. They are often on the defensive and compensate for their feelings of insecurity not by aggression but by anxiety, over-caution, and cowardice. Burdened by their insecurity, they constantly seek support.

Rajasika (restless and aggressive) persons are over-optimistic and self-aggrandizing. They often play the macho role to a ludicrous degree. They have inflated egos and are puffed up with pride, arrogance, and self-importance. In their persistent efforts to gain the upper hand, they make their lives a series of bloody battles. Tending to be vain, greedy, manipulative, domineering, jealous, and over-ambitious, they often exhibit schoolboy or schoolgirl behavior. At home, at work, and in society, they are anxious to win a point by their remarks, letting others know that they know better.

Sattvika (balanced) persons are neither aggressive nor defensive, neither optimistic nor pessimistic. They are temperate, moderate, pragmatic in human relations, integrated in their goals, and mature in their judgments. They have strong individualities that refuse to follow the crowd and are not easily swayed by mass opinion.

The characteristic traits of these categories are described by the Bhagavad Gita in the areas of a seeker's faith, sacrifice, austerity, and offerings.

Faith:

Men in whom *sattva* prevails worship the gods; men in whom *rajas* prevails worship demigods and demons; and men in whom *tamas* prevails worship ghosts and disembodied spirits.

Those vain and conceited men who, impelled by the force of their lust and attachment, subject themselves to severe austerities not ordained by the scriptures,

And, fools that they are, torture all their bodily organs, and Me [the Lord who is the witness of man's thoughts and deeds], too, who dwell within the body—know that they are fiendish in their resolves.

Sacrifice:

That sacrifice is of the nature of *sattva* which is offered according to the scriptural rules by those who expect no reward and who firmly believe that it is their duty to sacrifice.

But that sacrifice which is performed in expectation of reward and for the sake of ostentation—know that to be of the nature of *rajas.*

And that sacrifice which is not performed according to the scriptural rules, and in which no food is distributed, no hymns are chanted, and no fee paid, and which is devoid of faith, is said to be of the nature of *tamas.*

Austerity:

This threefold austerity [of the body, speech, and mind] practiced with supreme faith by steadfast men, without the desire for fruit, is said to be of the nature of *sattva.*

The austerity that is practiced in order to gain respect, honour, and reverence, and for ostentation, is said to be of the nature of *rajas*. Its result is uncertain and transitory.

The austerity that is practiced with a determination based on foolishness, by means of self-torture, or for the purpose of ruining another is declared to be of the nature of *tamas*.

Offerings:

That gift which is made to one who can make no return, and with the feeling that it is one's duty to give, and which is given at the right place and time and to a worthy person—such a gift is held to be of the nature of *sattva*.

But that which is given for the sake of recompense or with the expectation of fruit or in a grudging mood is accounted as of the nature of *rajas*.

And the gift that is made without respect or with disdain, at an improper place and time, and to an unworthy person is declared to be of the nature of *tamas*.[2]

The guna structure of a person is also revealed in his or her manners and conduct, choice of dress, religion, ethics, posture, and look.

The manners and conduct of a *sattvika* person in general are deep, enduring, steady, and true. While a *rajasika* person is over-enthusiastic, boisterous, fickle, and impatient and a *tamasika* person callous, careless, clumsy, and cold, a *sattvika* person is more calm and assured.

A *sattvika* person's dress is appropriate, clean, proportionate, aesthetic, and modest. The dress of a *rajasika* person is superfluous, colorful, and gaudy. A *tamasika* person's dress is characterized by slovenliness, uncleanliness, a lack of proportion, and a lack of any aesthetic sense whatsoever.

The ethical and religious ideal of a *sattvika* person is universal, tolerant, peaceful, sincere, and spontaneous. In contrast, a *rajasika* person tends to be self-righteous, aggressive, and hollow and a *tamasika* person narrow, superstitious, secretive, and influenced by the occult.

A *sattvika* person is calm and pleasing in posture, steady in look, and gentle in movement. A *rajasika* person will often be restless in posture, agitated in look, and noisy in movement and a *tamasika* person may stoop low in sitting, exhibit vacant eyes, a burdened face, and a lack of enthusiasm in movement.

If we want to understand a person or want to help someone, it is first necessary to determine the person's *guna* composition and then act accordingly. Each person must be handled individually as a unique personality. Friendship with a *sattvika* person requires one kind of expression, perhaps no external expression at all, whereas friendship with a *rajasika* person necessitates both expression and demonstration of the friendship. The same principle applies to business and other relationships. We can regulate our words, methods of expression, and system of application in keeping with the *guna* structure of the person we are dealing with.

Right behavior is *sattvika* behavior. Our behavior is the outcome of our attitude toward our inner being. Persons who have no respect for themselves cannot respect others. Persons cannot forgive others if they have not had the experience of being forgiven. Those who do not trust themselves are generally cynical and mistrustful of others.

Right behavior is disciplined behavior. It involves discipline of the body, including physical gestures and posture, of speech and of the mind, including thoughts, feelings, and attitudes. We must be aware that it is possible to hurt another person without speaking, just by our silence or posture. Our reactions and feelings can be detected in the emotional charge of words and expressions.

Right behavior calls for the practice of self-mastery. Self-mastery is exercising conscious control over our emotions, actions, and habits. Self-mastery is the key to all success, whether material or spiritual. The Bhagavad Gita asks us to practice three disciplines for self-mastery, also known as three austerities:

> Worship of the gods, of the twice-born, of teachers, and of the wise; cleanliness, uprightness, continence, and non-violence —these are said to be the austerity of the body.

> Words that do not give offence and that are truthful, pleasant, and beneficial, and also the regular recitation of the Vedas— these are said to be the austerity of speech.

> Serenity of mind, gentleness, silence, self-control, and purity of heart—these constitute the austerity of the mind.[3]

OBSTACLES TO RIGHT BEHAVIOR

The obstacles that stand in the way of right behavior are: narcissism, egotism, intolerance, insensitivity, oversensitivity, intoxication of power and wealth, emotional and intellectual immaturity, overcritical nature, rude tongue, and a holier-than-thou attitude.

Narcissism is a mental state in which persons lose contact with the everyday reality of the outside world. Narcissistic persons are so filled with themselves that others do not exist for them. Their value judgments, perceptions, and opinions are heavily prejudiced, and they rationalize their prejudices in one way or another. Narcissism distorts our capacity to think and judge in a rational way.

Egotism is different from narcissism. Narcissism implies an inability to perceive reality in all its fullness, while egotism implies little or no concern, love, or sympathy for others. Egotism makes persons extremely selfish. For egotists, the whole world consists of what happens to them and the way they feel. Like spoiled children, they insist on having everything their way. They want reciprocated love, success in their vocation, and the satisfaction of personal friendship but are thwarted in every attempt to get them by their extremely inflated self-importance. They relentlessly crave the admiration of others.

Egotistic persons are extremely sensitive to criticism. Anybody who does not agree with them is a fool. They love to be flattered and become furious when criticized. They live in a world of vast conspiracies. Even casual conversations of strangers on the street can trouble them greatly.

Intolerance is a great impediment to decent behavior. Intolerant people are dogmatic in their views and desperately try to impose those views on others. Tolerance is the first step toward harmonious human relations. The next step is acceptance. No abiding friendship or love can develop between two individuals unless they learn to accept their differences.

Insensitive persons try to live lives of pure reason. They look upon feeling and sentiment as human weaknesses. They fail to understand that life is often guided not by reason but by feeling. In a small village, there once lived a learned philosopher. Emotions and feelings had no meaning for him. He scrupulously observed the rules of literal truthfulness. An elderly woman of that village had two sons. Her first son died. She arranged a memorial service for her son and invited all the people of the village, including the philosopher, who said he would come. The philosopher, however, forgot the date and time of the service and failed to appear. After two weeks, he realized that he had not honored the invitation and felt disturbed at not having kept his word. So he went straight to the woman's house, profusely apologized, and said, "Madam, I am so sorry I could not come to your son's memorial service. But I promise you today that I will not forget again. I will definitely come when your next son dies."

Oversensitivity is another obstacle that prevents a person from having an objective view of others. A small word, an insignificant act, or petty difference of opinion can forever destroy a friendship. Too occupied with their own feelings and prejudices, over-sensitive persons perceive others with an emotionally charged vision. You can know a person only by being identified with that person, which calls for the capacity to detach yourself from your subjective preoccupations.

When people become *intoxicated by power and wealth*, they eventually forfeit the sympathy and goodwill of all and are forced to live in a world that is bitter and lonely. When such persons lose their power and position, flatterers and so-called friends do not hesitate to leave them. Warning us about the delusion of power and wealth, Shankaracharya writes:

> *Boast not of youth or friends or wealth;*
> *Swifter than eyes can wink, by Time*
> *Each of these is stolen away.*
> *Abjure the illusion of the world*
> *And join yourself to timeless Truth.*[4]

Emotional immaturity can take two forms: introversion or extroversion. Extreme introverts are unable to escape from their self-centered brooding and morbid mind. In extreme introversion, there is a repression of response to objective, external concerns. Extremely introverted persons lead self-enclosed lives. They think that all good things in life come from within themselves and withdraw from society. As they withdraw more and more into their private world, they experience a sense of alienation from the social environment. They begin to feel like strangers in their own world. They look upon society as deceptive, illusory, and feel bitterness within. Extreme extroverts, on the other hand, are outgoing and overreaching in their social relationships. But beneath their outgoing nature, they lead very shallow and superficial lives. They suffer from an alienation from the center of their being. They talk like heaven but feel like hell. They hide their inner emptiness and self-alienation under endless pretense and false optimism.

Intellectual immaturity is another obstacle to human relations. Despite numerous intellectual accomplishments, many persons remain unhappy, and their unhappiness becomes obvious in their manners and behavior. In company or conversation, they assume a bearing of authority and superiority. Whatever they say must be accepted as infallible, and whatever they do must be taken as perfect. To recognize and appreciate another person's worth and accomplishments is against their nature. Learning from others is beneath their dignity. Knowledge, which is supposed to make a person humble, makes them arrogant.

Persons of an *overcritical nature* are blind to the positive side of people, emphasizing only their negative side. They criticize anything they do not like. When differences with another person are not understood and accepted, great damage is inflicted upon the social relationship.

Many justify their *rude tongue* by claiming to be honest, forthright, and straightforward. They are often self-righteous and have little or no respect for the feelings of others. Donning the halo of a fanatical follower of truth, a rude person makes no allowances for human weakness. Such persons eventually find themselves lost in the wilderness of isolation. No one wants to hear them speak.

There are persons with a *holier-than-thou attitude* who are quick to brand others as unethical and unspiritual. They like to play the self-proclaimed role of social conscience and show great zeal in trying to change others. Highly opinionated, they pass judgment on others, even when such judgment is unasked for and unwanted. Mature people, however, expect from friends not empty advice but sympathy. In the absence of sympathy, mere advice becomes repulsive. Even good advice without sympathy sounds meaningless. We have the right to criticize others or correct others only when we love them and are willing to suffer and sacrifice for them.

ETHICAL BEHAVIOR AND BASIC VIRTUES

Right conduct is a spiritual obligation. It is the spiritual obligation of a person to give support to others, and that support must be given with respect, humility, and gratitude in order to fulfill the codes of ethical conduct. Ethical conduct finds its fulfillment in the realization of the spiritual oneness of existence. This realization alone can guarantee the total well-being of a person. Yoga and Vedanta offer five basic virtues, essential for ethical and spiritual well-being:

- *Ahimsa,* or non-violence, calls for not doing violence to others by thought, word, gesture, and action and for having goodwill for all.

- *Satya,* or veracity, implies being straightforward and truthful in speech. Such straightforwardness and truthfulness should be pleasant, and the motivation for being so should be doing good to others. Truthful speech that hurts or injures others ceases to be truthful.

- *Asteya,* or abstention from covetousness, consists not merely of abstaining from any outward act of theft but also of having inward freedom from greed and possessiveness.

- *Brahmacharya* has two aspects, observance and restraint. The observance aspect calls for dwelling on Brahman, the inmost Self of all beings, while restraint asks for control of the gross urges and abstention from lewdness in thought, speech, and action.

- *Aparigraha* is the practice of self-reliance and freedom from dependence.

Expressions of right behavior vary from one culture to another. Yet there are certain principles that are universal. The following sections provide guidelines for right behavior in conversation, friendship, and human relations in general.

Conversation

In regard to conversation, Swami Vivekananda tells us, "It is always good to tell a man his defects in a direct way and in a friendly spirit to make him convinced of them, so that he may correct himself—but you should trumpet forth his virtues before others."[5]

Conversation is more than talking. It is a social skill by which a person makes a cordial connection with another person. What is important in a conversation is not the formalities of a greeting or carefully scripted words of introduction but a sense of genuine interest in the other person. It is necessary to find out what the other person likes and dislikes and to respect his or her views. One must be courteous enough to give others the freedom to express their views.

Listen carefully and attentively to the other person. Listening has two aspects. One is listening through the ears. But listening is incomplete unless one has also learned to listen through the eyes. Listening through the eyes is carefully observing the facial expressions, gestures, postures, and body movements of the other person. This is listening between the words. Many times one can learn more from what the other person does not say than from what is said.

Learn to take responsibility for your mistakes. Apologizing for unintentional remarks is a mark of spiritual well-being. There are many who associate saying "I'm sorry" with submission or surrender. They fail to understand that accepting responsibility for behavioral lapses or unintentional mistakes is a mark of virtue and dignity.

Be your own self. Don't try to be someone you are not. When a person imitates another person's style, mannerisms, accents, gestures, and postures, he or she loses authenticity and appears phony and artificial. It adds another layer between us and our true Self.

Friendship

Know how to give. When you praise your friend, be generous in your praise and don't expect any return. Praise, do not flatter, your friend. Flattery is usually untrue and overstated. One also should not take the loyalty of a friend for granted. Such loyalty has to be appreciated and returned.

Accept a friend as he or she is. No one in this world is perfect. In accepting a friend, one must accept both the friend's good and bad qualities. Go out of your way to serve your friends with sincerity and be there when your friends need help. Seeing the same Self in your friends and yourself, rendering service to your friends in difficult times is the most tangible service to God.

Holy Mother Sri Sarada Devi gives us the essential meaning of friendship: "The purpose of one's life is fulfilled only when one is able to give joy to another."[6]

Human relations

In her last message, Holy Mother advised us: "My child, if you want peace, then do not look into anybody's faults. Look into your own faults. Learn to make the world your own. No one is a stranger, my child; the whole world is your own."[7]

Be judicious in your response. We often respond to a situation or person hastily. We make promises we cannot fulfill and give hope and assurances we cannot guarantee. It is therefore desirable to develop the habit of responding only after thinking of the pros and cons of a response.

Be tolerant. If you hope to get along with people, you must understand that you cannot always have your way. To give in is not to sacrifice the fundamental principle of honesty. It is meeting the other party halfway and compromising the nonessentials.

Do not cherish victory everywhere. Never cherish victory over your son, daughter, disciple, or teacher. In such cases, your defeat is your victory.

Never be influenced by others' opinions. Never hear through another's ears or see through another's eyes and thereby form your opinions. Depend upon your own direct verification of the facts before you act or react.

"Hiss but do not hurt." If you have a kind heart, you need a tough exterior to defend yourself. Sri Ramakrishna's advice is to keep on hissing, but not to hurt. He tells the story of a poisonous snake that received a sacred word from a holy man so that it would no longer do harm. It became so nonviolent and passive that when some cowherd boys picked it up and dashed it repeatedly on the ground, it could not show any anger. Later, when the holy man returned and saw the snake's pitiable condition, he scolded it and said, "What a shame! You are such a fool! You don't know how to protect yourself. I asked you not to bite, but I did not forbid you to hiss. Why didn't you scare them by hissing?"[8] Sri Ramakrishna says:

> A man living in society should make a show of anger to protect himself from evil-minded people. But he should not harm anybody in anticipation of harm likely to be done him.[9]

> God undoubtedly dwells in the hearts of all—righteous and unrighteous; but a man should not have dealings with the unholy, the wicked, the impure. He must not be intimate with them. With some of them he may exchange words, but with others he shouldn't go even that far. He should keep aloof from such people.[10]

CONCLUSION

It may be asked why a person should be decent to everyone. Is it good to squander one's decency on those who do not deserve it? May not goodness showered on the wicked be taken as weakness? In answer to these questions, the sages and saints of all traditions have affirmed that goodness is the inherent nature of good persons, and they cannot behave otherwise. Good persons are good because they can put up with the bad behavior of bad persons. It is beneath their dignity to come down to the level of the bad.

A classical story describes how good persons behave even when their goodness goes unappreciated: A holy man once lived in seclusion on the bank of a river. One day he noticed that a scorpion had fallen into the water. Out of kindness, he picked it up with his hand to save it. The scorpion, in turn, stung the holy man. Writhing in pain, the holy man dropped the scorpion on the ground. A little later, the scorpion again fell into the water, again the holy man rescued it, and again it stung him badly. A third time the same thing happened. A person standing nearby asked the holy man, "Sir, why are you doing this again and again? Don't you know, sir, that a scorpion never gives up its habit of stinging?" The holy man replied, "If the scorpion does not give up its habit of stinging, why should I give up my habit of doing good?"

8

Truthfulness: Its Practice and Its Dilemmas

Truthfulness is the foundation of all morality. Moral conduct is indispensable not only for spiritual welfare but also for material and psychological fulfillment. Adherence to morality ensures a person's health, happiness, and peace of mind. The Sanskrit word for health, *swastha*, means "being true to one's Self." A person's real strength is strength of mind, and such strength is based upon a moral foundation.

The problems of human life are more psychological and spiritual than biological. The two prerequisites for the enjoyment of life—a sound body and a sound mind—can be attained only through the practice of moral virtues. No decent life is possible where dishonesty and deception prevail. Moral fitness gives us a voice of truth that carries power. It lets us see the interrelatedness of all life and the oneness of existence and inspires us to feel and act for the welfare of others.

The core of all moral fitness is truthfulness—the unmistakable mark of a pure heart, the source of all strength, power, and inspiration. Truthfulness is the very heart of spirituality. God as Ultimate Reality is the truth of all truths, and all that is required of a person to walk in the path of God is truthfulness. The goal of life is self-fulfillment through Self-knowledge. Truth is self-evident and carries its own credentials, but we fail to perceive the truth because of the impurities of the mind. The aim of all spiritual practice is to purify the mind.

Spiritual practices consist of prayer, contemplation, meditation, and chanting of the sacred word, all of which are regulatory. The mind, however, cannot be regulated unless it has been brought under control, and to attain such control, the practice of moral virtues is vital. Moral practices endow a spiritual seeker with a steel frame foundation upon which the spiritual structure can be raised. Spiritual practice without moral purity is counterproductive and dangerous. An ancient proverb says, "If you feed a cobra milk and honey without taking out its poisonous fangs, it will only produce poison." The practice of moral virtues aims to remove the poisonous fangs of the mind.

The practice of moral virtues is common to all systems of thought. These virtues are truthfulness, nonviolence, noncovetousness, dispassion, discrimination, control over the mind and the senses, fortitude, faith, and tranquility of the mind. Among these, truthfulness leads the way. Because God is the embodiment of all truth, one who holds to truth holds to God. Truthfulness is the greatest purifier, the highest austerity, and the very backbone of all morality.

THE DILEMMA OF TRUTHFULNESS

The question is often asked, "Is it possible for a person to be truthful under all circumstances?" There are occasions when a truthful person is tormented by certain moral dilemmas. As Sissela Bok in *Lying: Moral Choice in Public and Private Life* writes:

> Should physicians lie to dying patients to delay the fear and anxiety which the truth might bring them? Should professors exaggerate the excellence of their students on recommendations in order to give them a better chance in a tight job market? Should parents conceal from children the fact that they were adopted? Should social scientists send investigators

masquerading as patients to physicians in order to learn about racial and sexual biases in diagnoses and treatment? Should government lawyers lie to congressmen who might otherwise oppose a much-needed welfare bill? And should journalists lie to those from whom they seek information in order to expose corruption?[1]

There are also other dilemmas. In correspondence and social exchanges, people often use expressions such as "It is good to see you," "Very truly yours," and "Yours sincerely." These are polite expressions and used widely for cordial human relationships in everyday life. Even though they may not always be sincere and true, these expressions are accepted by society as necessary lies to be tolerated for human understanding and good neighborliness. From the point of view of truthfulness, should we refrain from using these words and expressions in verbal exchanges, even though telling the truth in such circumstances would run the risk of being unsocial, impolite, and unkind? It is said that a lawyer was once administering the oath to a witness. The lawyer asked, "Do you swear to tell the truth, the whole truth, and nothing but the truth, so help you God?" The witness replied, "If I could tell the truth, the whole truth, and nothing but the truth, *then I would be God!*" The witness's response is honest, true, and speaks for the vast majority of people.

Truth is stranger than fiction in a world where selfishness, greed, and hypocrisy rule. Moral values and principles are widely compromised for the sake of material gain. Hypocrisy is often practiced under the guise of social responsibility. Telling a lie is frequently justified with an intelligent excuse, such as "the end justifies the means"; that is, dishonest means are justified in the interest of the benefit attained. The end result of this laxness in the definition of a lie has been spiritual anemia in our individual lives and in society.

Truth-telling is natural and spontaneous; lying has to be learned. When children start telling lies, they lose their innocence, and become secretive. A person who lives on lies is haunted by a sense of guilt, anxiety, and restlessness. There is the story of a person who, after filing his tax return with the IRS, came to realize that he had not listed all his income on the tax form and therefore had not paid enough taxes. Overcome with guilt, he wrote a letter to the IRS:

> Gentlemen:
>
> I am sorry to inform you that I discovered I did not list all my income on the tax form, and since then I am unable to sleep. Please find enclosed a check for $150.00. If I still cannot sleep, I will send you the rest.

We instinctively feel lying to be undesirable, yet cannot give it up.

TRUTHFULNESS AND THE SACRED TRADITIONS

Whatever may be the predicaments and the dilemmas, a spiritual seeker cannot afford to make any compromise with truth. Why is truthfulness so vital for spiritual life? First, it is the most vital teaching of every spiritual tradition. Jesus calls Satan the father of the lie. The lie is primarily the denial of God. In Dante's *Inferno,* liars are tormented in the eighth circle of hell, lowest of all except for that inhabited by traitors. "Thou hatest all the workers of iniquity; thou wilt destroy all that speak a lie" (Psalms 5:5–6).

Two beliefs often support the rigid rejection of all lies: that God rules out all lies, and that God will punish those who lie. Kant says, "By a lie a man throws away and, as it were, annihilates his dignity as a man."[2] St. Augustine takes a firm stand against all lies. His definition leaves no room at all for justifiable falsehood. In contrast, St. Thomas Aquinas "set a pattern that is still followed by Catholic theologians. He distinguished three kinds of lies: the officious, or helpful, lies; the jocose lies, told in jest; and the mischievous, or malicious, lies told to harm someone. Only the latter constitute mortal sin for Aquinas. He agreed with Augustine that all lies are sin, but regarded the officious and jocose lies as less serious."[3]

The Talmud gives "three exceptions to the rule of truthfulness ... : 'tractate,' 'bed,' and 'hospitality.' *Tractate* is explained by the commentaries to mean that if a scholar is asked if he is familiar with a certain portion of the Talmud he may, from modesty, untruthfully say that he is ignorant. An untruth is permitted if its aim is the avoidance of a parade of learning. *Bed* is understood to mean that if a scholar is asked questions concerning his marital relations he may give an untruthful answer. *Hospitality* is understood to mean that a scholar who had been generously treated by his host may decide not to tell the truth about his reception if he fears that as a result the host may be embarrassed by unwelcome guests. In addition, there is a general principle of the Talmud that where peace demands it a lie may be told."[4]

THE VEDANTA VIEW OF TRUTHFULNESS

Vedanta considers truthfulness as the foundation of all moral virtues. Emphasizing the need for truthfulness, Sri Ramakrishna says:

> Truthfulness in speech is the *tapasya* [austerity] of the Kaliyuga [modern age]. It is difficult to practise other austerities in this cycle. By adhering to truth one attains God. Tulsidas said: "Truthfulness, obedience to God, and the regarding of others' wives as one's mother, are the greatest virtues. If one does not realise God by practising them, then Tulsidas is a liar."[5]
>
> God cannot be realized without guilelessness.
>
> *Cherish love within your heart;*
> *abandon cunning and deceit:*
> *Through service, worship, selflessness,*
> *does Rama's blessed vision come.*

> Even those engaged in worldly activities, such as office work
> or business, should hold to the truth. Truthfulness alone is
> the discipline in the Kaliyuga.[6]

If a person clings tenaciously to truth, he or she ultimately realizes God. Without this regard for truth, one gradually loses everything.[7] Swami Vivekananda says, "Practise truthfulness. Twelve years of absolute truthfulness in thought, word, and deed gives a man what he wills. Be chaste in thought, word, and action. Chastity is the basis of all religions."[8] Swami Turiyananda, a direct disciple of Sri Ramakrishna, says, "Truth is God. Falsehood is maya. One gets everything by holding on to truth."[9]

Truthfulness embodies three essential guidelines. First, the object must be correctly apprehended by the speaker's mind; there should not be any illusion or error. Second, there should be no intentional deceit, indulgence, or vagueness with regard to the fact presented by speech. Veracity precludes half-truths, evasions, and subterfuges, all of which are to be treated as lies. Third, speech must be conducive to the welfare of all beings. Even the most precise speech falls short of veracity if not spoken for the good of all. When truthful speech becomes a cause of pain, suffering, or injury to any living creature, it is not to be regarded as truthfulness. Even to recount another person's real faults, when it serves no good purpose, is considered untruthful.

There are, however, circumstances where truth is considered falsehood, and falsehood truth. For example, a murderer pursuing someone should not be told the truth of that person's whereabouts; if silence would arouse the murderer's suspicion, telling a lie would be appropriate. If rigid adherence to truthfulness is likely to do more harm than good, the evil should be averted by telling a lie if necessary. Again, speech must be agreeable and pleasant. Unpleasant truth-telling must be avoided by all means. Under such circumstances, one is advised to keep silent, plead ignorance, or leave the place. The practice of truthfulness requires strict avoidance of all exaggerations, equivocations, and pretenses.

Vedanta considers truthfulness from the spiritual point of view, as opposed to the points of view of utilitarian or scientific ethics. Utilitarian ethics aims to secure the maximum utility for a society; scientific ethics, largely influenced by biology, holds that whatever is conducive to the survival of a particular individual or species is good for it. The absolute necessity for a spiritual seeker to lead a perfectly truthful life follows from the very nature of Ultimate Reality, which guides the laws of the universe and our individual lives. The Upanishads designate Ultimate Reality as the true Self of all. This Self is the truth of all truths, the bond of all bonds of unity, the basis of all love and harmony:

> There is One who is the eternal Reality among non-eternal objects, the one [truly] conscious Entity among conscious objects, and who, though non-dual, fulfils the desires of many. Eternal peace belongs to the wise, who perceive Him within themselves—not to others.[10]

> Truth alone prevails, not falsehood. By truth the path is laid out, the Way of the Gods, on which the seers, whose every desire is satisfied, proceed to the Highest Abode of the True.[11]

A seeker aspiring to perceive this Reality must follow the laws of Reality. Anything that violates the law of truth also violates the laws of love and harmony and prevents one from reaching the spiritual goal of God-realization.

Psychologically, untruthfulness in its various forms creates all kinds of unnecessary complications in our lives and becomes a source of constant mental disturbance. According to Swami Brahmananda, the eminent disciple of Sri Ramakrishna, "To tell a lie is the greatest sin. A drunkard or a man who frequents houses of ill fame may be trusted, but never a liar! It is the blackest of sins."[12] For deluded persons, lying is one of the simplest and easiest means of escaping an undesirable situation or difficulty. They are unable to see that by avoiding one difficulty they create many others of a more serious nature. Those who keep a watchful eye on their thoughts and actions notice that a lie usually requires a number of other lies for its support, and that in spite of all their efforts, circumstances often take such an unexpected turn that the lie is exposed sooner or later. This effort to maintain falsehoods and false appearances causes a peculiar strain in our subconscious mind and provides a congenial soil for all kinds of emotional disturbances, such as fear, anxiety, and guilt.

Practice of truthfulness is vital for spiritual advancement. As we advance along the path, which is a journey through the layers of the unconscious, we confront many problems, to which solutions cannot be found either in reference books or in rational thinking. The only means at our disposal to solve such problems is an unclouded intuition. Nothing clouds the intuition more than untruthfulness—gross or subtle, direct or indirect. Seekers who begin their spiritual quest without first acquiring the virtue of truthfulness are like persons walking in the darkness of night without light. Having nothing to guide them in their difficulties, they are sure to be lost in the wilderness of the illusions that stand in their way. That is why seekers are asked to put on the armor of perfect truthfulness in thought, word, and deed, so that they can make their way to the goal.

9
The True Friend

Truthfulness is the basis of all friendship. We must know that our best friends are those who help us in our spiritual quest for Truth.

Friendship is vital for our survival, sustenance, and well-being. We need friends for consolation in grief and support in distress, for self-expression and sharing joy. Life is interdependent, not independent. Interdependence is not just a matter of religious idealism—it is reality. The human body is molded out of the physical universe; its cells are derived from parents' bodies; its food is gathered from the vegetable and animal worlds. The individual mind is part of the universal mind. We are indebted to fellow human beings for their sympathy in times of hardship and to the sages and saints for moral and spiritual inspiration. The universe is one single organism, in which there is no gap between atom, cell, sense, self, and society. This oneness of existence is the basis for all ethics and morality.

The human individual is essentially a social being. Relatedness—the feeling of belonging to a larger whole and of being of value to others—is a natural necessity of life. A person needs to express love and sympathy for others and wants to receive the same from them. He or she cannot satisfy the urge for love without being socially conscious. A person seeks companions for emotional support and feels lonely when no one is around. Rick Weiss of *National Geographic Magazine* writes:

> Gerontologists are just starting to appreciate the ways that social and psychological factors can contribute to the quality of life in old age, and even to longevity. Studies have shown that seniors who have emotional support from friends and family have lower levels of stress hormones circulating in their blood and are less likely to die in the near future than are those who feel lonely and isolated. Scientists don't know all the ways that emotions and attitudes influence physical health. But health does seem to be enhanced by giving and sharing.[1]

Self-expression is not to be identified with the sex instinct, the desire for power, or the drive for self-preservation. Vedanta maintains that the instinct for self-expression stems from a deep longing for self-expansion. As Swami Vivekananda says, "Expansion is life; contraction is death. Love is life, and hatred is death."[2] Suppression of the instinct for self-expression can derange a person's mind. When persons are forced to live in isolation against their will, without friends or companions, they tend to become unbalanced, if not insane.

We are influenced psychologically by our friends and relatives, and in the same way, we influence them. This fact calls upon us to become free, good-natured, and cooperative. Too few of us realize that the law of gravity is to the stars as the law of relatedness is to human beings, and that attraction and repulsion are to space as approval and rejection are to human society.

The primary joy of life comes from the acceptance, approval, and companionship of our neighbors and friends. When we are appreciated and needed by those who know us, we get the first taste of peace and self-satisfaction. Devoid of friendship and fellowship, a person becomes irrelevant in this universe, running from loneliness to loneliness.

MARKS OF A TRUE FRIEND

True friendship is utterly selfless. To care for a person implies feeling responsible for his or her total well-being—not just physical existence. Such friendship is an active concern, not mere passive cordiality.

True friendship is tolerant. Tolerance is the positive effort to understand another's beliefs, practices, and habits. True friendship between two persons honors and leaves intact the freedom of individuality. Voltaire's dictum, "I do not agree with a word that you say, but I will defend to the death your right to say it,"[3] is for all ages and places the perfect utterance of the ideal of tolerance. When we force our friends to conform to our convictions, we violate their rights.

True friendship is always honest and sincere. As Emerson says in his essay "Friendship":

> A friend is a person with whom I may be sincere. Before him I may think aloud. I am arrived at last in the presence of a man so real and equal that I may drop even those most undermost garments of dissimulation, courtesy, and second thought, which men never put off, and may deal with him with the simplicity and wholeness with which one chemical atom meets another.[4]

In true friendship, there is no place for fear. Fear in friendship comes only when there is a selfish motive. A true friend will always trust you; you won't have to prove yourself in order to hold his or her loyal friendship. A true friend will never say anything behind your back that would not be said to you in person.

The most enduring foundation of true friendship is the spiritual kinship between two persons. A true friend is one who not only wishes us well here but also hereafter. Such a friend inspires us in the path of God, protects us from vices and temptations, intercedes on our behalf with God, and prays for our spiritual welfare. On the other hand, the person who makes us forget God and arouses in our mind worldly propensities can never be called a true friend—no matter how pleasant or likable that person may be.

True friendship cannot be taken for granted. It is like a plant that requires nurturing and caring, without which it withers and dies. Human nature is often frivolous, and human greed seems to have no limit. Self-interest is pervasive and human ingratitude endemic. The heart that is now full of love may become full of jealousy later. In politics, it is said that there is no such thing as permanent friendship or permanent enmity but only permanent interest. Business friendships, similarly, are all out of self-interest. In social exchanges, friendship is a matter of convenience. Most so-called friends are fair-weather friends who gather around a person in good times to flatter and cheer but who vanish when that person meets with difficulty. Self-serving and insincere, they remain friends as long as their self-interest lasts. With their worldly propensities and craftiness, such friends prove to be the enemies of a person in the spiritual path. In all countries at all times, the company of such worldly friends has been the cause of moral and spiritual downfall for seekers of God. The Bhagavad Gita graphically describes how slowly and silently this downfall occurs:

> When a man dwells on objects, he feels an attachment for them. Attachment gives rise to desire, and desire breeds anger.

> From anger comes delusion; from delusion, the failure of memory; from the failure of memory, the ruin of discrimination; and from the ruin of discrimination the man perishes.[5]

There is nothing more ruinous to a person than the company of a bad friend. According to the *Narada Bhakti Sutras*, bad company is the breeding ground of all sins and vices, "because it causes lust, wrath, delusion, loss of memory, loss of reason, and, finally, total wreck of the man."[6] Bad company fans the flames of passion. "These propensities, though at first like ripples, acquire the proportions of a sea, by reason of bad company."[7] In his last message, Sri Krishna says:

> A mental wave is never produced by anything that has not been seen or heard. So the mind of a man who controls his senses is gradually stilled and is perfectly at peace.... Thus the wise man should shun evil company and associate with the holy. It is these who by their words take away the attachment of the mind.[8]

These are the cold, hard facts of life, however unpleasant and pessimistic they may appear. True friendship is, indeed, rare. So Swami Vivekananda says:

> In happiness, in misery, in famine, in pain, in the grave, in heaven, or in hell, who never gives me up is my friend. Is such friendship a joke? A man may have salvation through such friendship.[9]

THE GREATEST FRIEND

The spiritual journey toward God-consciousness or Self-knowledge is essentially a solitary one, on which no one can help us but ourselves and our own mind. Our greatest friends are those who remind us of this truth and who inspire us to attain love of God and awareness of the Self. True friends encourage us to depend on no one but God. Sri Ramakrishna conveys this message in the following song:

> *Remember this, O mind! Nobody is your own;*
> *Vain is your wandering in this world.*
> *Trapped in the subtle snare of maya as you are,*
> *Do not forget the [Divine] Mother's name.*
>
> *Only a day or two men honour you on earth*
> *As lord and master; all too soon*

That form, so honoured now, must needs be cast away,
When Death, the Master, seizes you.

Even your beloved wife, for whom, while yet you live,
You fret yourself almost to death,
Will not go with you then; she too will say farewell,
And shun your corpse as an evil thing.[10]

The same message is repeated by the Master:

True knowledge makes one feel: "O God, You alone do everything. You alone are my own. And to You alone belong houses,
buildings, family, relatives, friends, the whole world. All is
Yours." But ignorance makes one feel: "I am doing everything.
I am the doer. House, buildings, family, children, friends, and
property are all mine."[11]

The following story strikingly illustrates who our only true
friends are: In a small village, there lived a pious man, virtuous and
honest. One day he received a summons from the king to appear
before him for judgment. The king was known for his eccentric-
ity and cruelty. The pious man became very much disturbed and
afraid. He had never done anything wrong or unjust, and so he
wondered how he could receive a summons like this.

The pious man had three friends: his best friend, his next best
friend, and his least intimate friend. He went to his best friend, explained his fear and distress, and asked him to come with him to
the king's court. His best friend, standing inside the front door of
his house, heard the whole matter and said, "I am afraid I cannot
accompany you to the king's court. I can only say good luck to you,
my friend," and he closed the door in his friend's face. The pious
man became terribly disappointed to realize that one whom he had
always regarded as his best friend would desert him at this time.

He then went to see his next best friend, told him the whole
problem, and made the same request of him. This friend said, "I
know you to be a good man, and you could not have done anything wrong. I'll come with you up to the palace gate, but I do not

intend to enter the palace and stand before the king. The king is unpredictable and may decide to put me in jail along with you." The pious man became disappointed for the second time.

Sad at heart and disillusioned about human nature, he went to his least intimate friend, from whom he never expected any help. When this third friend heard of his problem, this friend said to him: "I know you are an honest man and am certain that you are incapable of doing anything wrong. Do not worry, my friend. I will go before you to the court of the king and testify to him about your honesty and goodness." The pious man was greatly surprised at this pledge of support from a friend to whom he had never paid much attention.

The pious man in the story represents the human individual in distress; the king represents death, and the summons, the call of death. The palace gate stands for the graveyard. The "best friend" represents money and possessions. They say good-bye to a person at death and never come out of the house to accompany him. The "next best friend" represents family and friends. They accompany as far as the graveyard and then leave. The "least intimate friend" is the memory of one's good deeds, performed with selflessness for the benefit of others. The memory of good deeds becomes one's sole support in the fearful and solitary journey hereafter. Such a memory is a true and trusted friend. The memory of a good deed is like the messenger of truth that escorts the soul to the realm of Truth. The Bhagavad Gita declares this fact and says:

> In this [selfless action] no effort is ever lost and no harm is ever done. Even very little of this dharma [selfless action] saves a man from the Great Fear.[12]

A spiritual seeker proceeding along the spiritual path must understand the fact that there is a difference between spiritual friendship and social friendship. Living in the world calls for us to be friendly to all, but in our heart of hearts, we must know that our goal is God-realization and that anybody who helps us to realize this goal is our only true friend.

PART THREE

The Milestones

10

Signposts of Progress

The spiritual quest is a journey toward the goal of direct experience of Reality. There are four stages of development for the aspirant in this journey: inquiring, seeking, knowing, and seeing. The aspirant first inquires about truth, reads various scriptures, visits temples, and becomes associated with different traditions. In the second stage, the inquirer becomes a seeker. The seeker is no longer satisfied with information about, or roadmaps to, the goal and no longer searches for God or truth outside in temples or mountains, in sanctuaries or holy places. The seeker becomes committed to a path and an ideal, practices spiritual disciplines and discovers that to see God everywhere and in everything, he or she first needs to see God within. At the third stage, the seeker becomes a knower of Truth. In the depths of contemplation and meditation, the seeker begins to see the God within himself or herself. The seeker gains certainty of faith and begins to taste the bliss of the Divine. Yet the seeker's knowledge of the Divine, or God, is incomplete. Knowledge becomes complete only when the seeker is able to see the same God with eyes open and dedicate himself or herself to the service of God in all. As the Bhagavad Gita says, "He who, having been established in oneness, worships Me dwelling in all beings—that yogi, in whatever way he leads his life, lives in Me."[1]

In this regard, Sri Ramakrishna says:

He who has merely heard of milk is "ignorant." He who has
seen milk has "knowledge [*jnana*]." But he who has drunk
milk and been strengthened by it has attained vijnana.*[2]

The stages from seeking God to seeing God constitute an inward journey through the three states of our consciousness—
waking, dream, and dreamless sleep. Our only companion on this
journey is our mind—a mind that is unpredictable, changing, and
susceptible to delusion and temptations.

The road signs on this journey are not always clear. The dangers are many. Our mind so often deludes and ambushes us. More
often than not, our attachments pass as duty, our depression as
dispassion, escapism as self-surrender, callousness as detachment,
passing sentiments as devotion, cynicism as reason, regression as
progress, emotionalism as ecstasy, quantity as quality, occult phenomena as spiritual phenomena, rootlessness as universality, non-
commitment to any path as freedom, and fanaticism as
orthodoxy. It is vital to know that we are not lost, distracted, or
stalled on the path. We need to know where we stand, whether
we are overdoing or underachieving, and how far from the goal
we are.

TESTS OF PROGRESS

Sacred texts and traditions give us a number of tests of self-
evaluation for our guidance. Each of these markers may be experienced directly by one on a spiritual quest. They are common on
the Yoga and Vedanta path but are not exclusive to it.

Jnana is knowledge by which one is aware of one's identity with God.
Vijnana is special knowledge of God by which one sees the universe as the
manifestation of God.

Mystical experiences

The sacred word Om [Aum] is the primordial sound from which all other sounds emerge. It underlies all phonetic creations. The sounds of different languages and dialects are the various modifications of the primordial sound Om. Om embraces all levels of existence from the grossest to the finest. It signifies the correlation between the microcosm and macrocosm in all aspects. The three letters A, U, and M represent respectively the gross, the subtle, and the causal aspects of the Cosmic Being. The silence in which the sound merges represents the Pure Being underlying the three aspects. No other word conveys the significance of the Ultimate Reality as profoundly as the word Om. It is thus the most all-inclusive and most potent name of God.

At one stage, the seeker advancing along the spiritual path begins to hear the *anahata* sound, or Om, the uninterrupted sound of the universe. This indicates that the mind has reached the fourth center of consciousness, which is in the heart and called *anahata*.* Through the mind's eye, he or she sees fireflies and fog and hears the distant peal of bells. The sacred texts of Vedanta describe:

> When yoga is practiced, the forms which appear first and which gradually manifest Brahman are those of snow-flakes, smoke, sun, wind, fire, fire-flies, lightning, crystal, and the moon.[3]

> [The Anahata sound] is a spontaneous sound constantly going on by itself. It is the sound of the Pranava, Om. It originates in the Supreme Brahman [Supreme Reality] and is heard by

---

*According to the Yoga scriptures, there are six subtle centers of consciousness located in our spinal column. The first center is located at the base of the spine, the second at the base of the organ of generation, the third in the region of the navel, the fourth at the level of the heart, the fifth in the throat, and the sixth in between the eyebrows.

yogis. People immersed in worldliness do not hear it. A yogi alone knows that this sound originates both from his navel and from the Supreme Brahman.[4]

The powers of clairvoyance and clairaudience also come to the seeker, by which he or she can see and hear through the mind itself. The seeker experiences the rising of inner consciousness (kundalini). If the mind reaches the fourth center, the world appears to the seeker to be divine. The seeker sees light and says, "What is this? What is this?"

When the mind reaches the fifth center of consciousness in the throat, the seeker speaks only of God and nothing else; upon reaching the sixth center, the mind becomes silent in the total absorption of God-consciousness; and upon reaching the crown of the head, attains to the highest *samadhi*. The taste of intense bliss of this last state does not allow the seeker to ever return to outer consciousness.

The problem with mystical experiences as a test of progress, however, is that they are private and subjective. They can be temporary, false, a result of hallucination, autosuggestion, or heightened imagination. Their appearance may be sudden, stumbled upon, untimely, or a result of the weakness of the aspirant's nerves. They are not always sure indicators of spiritual progress.

Transformation of personality

Spiritual progress brings good health, good voice, increased efficiency, a lesser need of secrecy, experience of spiritual joy, and a spirit of self-dedication. These objective signs are dependable indicators of a seeker's spiritual progress. So-called transformation at the spiritual level without prior transformation at the physical and mental levels is always suspect.

Spiritual priorities

This is the test of the seeker's longing for the Divine. Every person has a list of priorities—material, psychological, and spiritual.

As a seeker progresses on the path toward the Divine, his or her priorities begin to change. The goal is to make God our number one priority and make all others subordinate to that priority.

Progress is measured in terms of the change in our priorities. When Self-realization becomes the number one priority, all our other goals—material and psychological—are subordinated to that goal.

Devotion

Devotion is the commitment of the heart. It gives spiritual nourishment to the soul. Progress in devotion is measured by the stage of devotion the seeker has attained. The first stage is *nishtha,* which is absolute loyalty to one spiritual ideal known in Yoga and Vedanta as the *Ishtadevata,* or Chosen Ideal. *Nishtha* brings *bhakti,* or devotion. Then, *bhakti* culminates in the stage of *bhava.* In this stage, the seeker experiences three moods: *vajjadasa,* when the seeker sings, dances, and chants the name of God; *ardhavaj-jadasa,* when the seeker uninterruptedly meditates on the Divine and becomes silent; and *antardasa,* the state of total absorption in the Divine. Higher than bhava is *mahabhava*—the highest stage of devotion. The seeker at this stage remains merged in *bhavasamadhi* all the time. Sri Ramakrishna explains a seeker's progress in devotion:

> How can a devotee attain [pure] love? First, the company of holy men. That awakens sraddha, faith in God. Then comes nishtha, single-minded devotion to the Ideal. In that stage the devotee does not like to hear anything but talk about God. He performs only those acts that please God. After nishtha comes bhakti, devotion to God; then comes bhava. Next mahabhava, then prema [divine love], and last of all the attainment of God Himself.[5]

Again, the stages of devotion have been classified as the following: The first stage is the life of law. At this stage, the seeker practices devotion as a discipline. The second stage is the life of love, when the seeker gradually develops loving attachment to the Ishtadevata and practices devotion out of pure love. The third stage is the life of divine inebriation, when the seeker in practicing devotion feels intoxicated with divine fervor. The fourth stage is the life of absorption. At this stage, the seeker communes with the Ishtadevata in silence and remains ever absorbed in this communion. The fifth stage is the life of self-dedication, when the seeker practices devotion for the welfare of all beings.

The quality of devotion is also an indicator of progress. The first qualitative stage of devotion is *sadharani,* when the seeker prays for the fulfillment of desires. The second stage is *samanjasa,* when the seeker practices devotion for his or her own pleasure and for the pleasure of the Ishtadevata. Then the seeker reaches the stage of *samartha,* when the seeker practices devotion only for the pleasure of the Chosen Ideal. Regarding the three kinds of love, Sri Ramakrishna says:

> There are [three] kinds of love: sadharani, samanjasa, and samartha. In the first, which is ordinary love, the lover seeks his own happiness; he doesn't care whether the other person is happy or not…. In the second, which is a compromise, both seek each other's happiness. This is a noble kind of love. But the third is the highest of all. Such a lover says to his beloved, "Be happy yourself, whatever may happen to me." Radha had this highest love. She was happy in Krishna's happiness.[6]

The attainment of true devotion must be matched by the attainment of knowledge. Knowledge teaches us that the Ishtadevata alone is our own, now and always. The Ishtadevata alone is our support, sustenance, and salvation. This knowledge alone can inspire a person toward God. When devotion is not supported by this knowledge, it is cheap sentiment. And when devotion does not inspire a person toward self-dedication, it is not considered genuine.

Four stages of advancement

There are four stages of a seeker's spiritual progress: beginner, struggling, adept, and perfect. Sri Ramakrishna describes:

> According to a certain school of thought there are four classes of devotees: the pravartaka [beginner], the sadhaka [aspiring], the siddha [perfect], and the siddha of the siddha [supremely perfect]. He who has just begun religious life is a pravartaka. Such a man puts his denominational marks on his body and forehead, wears a rosary around his neck, and scrupulously follows other outer conventions. The sadhaka has advanced farther. His desire for outer show has become less. He longs for the realization of God and prays to Him sincerely. He repeats the name of God and calls on Him with a guileless heart. Now, whom should we call the siddha? He who has the absolute conviction that God exists and is the sole Doer; he who has seen God. And who is the siddha of the siddha? He who has not merely seen God, but has intimately talked with Him as Father, Son, or Beloved.[7]

A beginner is one who has just stepped onto the spiritual path and tries to follow spiritual practice as sincerely as possible. Practice in this stage is mostly a discipline. The second stage is that of a struggling seeker. There is a struggle between the seeker's old tendencies, desires, and aspirations and the new tendencies, desires, and aspirations. In spiritual practice, he or she sometimes feels inspired and is sometimes taken over by the old tendencies. It is a common experience that just as the seeker begins to practice prayer, meditation, and *japa*, the mind resists. The mind, the seeker feels, is more turbulent than ever before. Swami Vivekananda describes this anxiety:

> The first lesson, then, is to sit for some time and let the mind run on. The mind is bubbling up all the time. It is like that monkey jumping about. Let the monkey jump as much as he can; you simply wait and watch. Knowledge is power, says the

proverb, and that is true. Until you know what the mind is doing you cannot control it. Give it the rein. Many hideous thoughts may come into it; you will be astonished that it was possible for you to harbour such thoughts; but you will find that each day the mind's vagaries are becoming less and less violent, that each day it is becoming calmer. In the first few months you will find that the mind has a great many thoughts; later you will find that they have somewhat decreased, and in a few more months they will be fewer and fewer, until at last the mind is under perfect control.[8]

The third stage is that of the perfect. The perfect seeker gains mastery over the mind, emotions, and moods, can invoke the spiritual mood at will, and is assured of his or her spiritual destiny. The fourth stage is the perfect. A supremely perfect seeker always remains mounted on yoga, remaining high in spiritual altitude. The supremely perfect seeker's mood for meditation and prayer follows him or her everywhere irrespective of situation and circumstance. The supremely perfect seeker gets glimpses of the Divine and remains established in the state of ethereal spiritual bliss.

Spiritual attainments

Yoga and Vedanta mention *siddhis,* or spiritual attainments, such as mantra *siddhi, vak siddhi, dhyana siddhi,* and *samadhi siddhi.*

By attaining mantra *siddhi,* a seeker feels that the Ishtamantra is more than words, often sees the mantra appearing in letters of fire in the mind, and feels that the mantra is following him or her everywhere as a constant companion and guide. The mantra repeats itself, bubbling up from within. By attaining *vak siddhi,* whatever the seeker says comes to be true. By practicing truthfulness in thought, word, and deed for twelve years—according to another view, twenty-eight years—the seeker attains this *siddhi.*

Dhyana siddhi is perfection in meditation. It is a state in which meditation pursues the seeker. The seeker does not have to make any effort. Swami Vivekananda was born with *dhyana siddhi.* Before going to bed, he would see a ball of light in front of him; then the ball would burst. He would be flooded with divine light. As a young man, he thought that perhaps everyone went to sleep with this experience. But when he asked his friends about it, he came to know that none of them experienced anything like it. When he told Sri Ramakrishna about this phenomenon, Sri Ramakrishna described it as a mark of *dhyana siddhi,* or perfection in meditation.

By attaining *samadhi siddhi,* the seeker is taken over by the state of *samadhi,* experiencing communion with the Divine. The seeker is established in the state of *samadhi* by the repeated experience of *samadhi.* Shankaracharya tells us that experiencing the state of *samadhi* once is not enough. One must experience *samadhi* repeatedly and get established in this state.

> Established in the ethereal plane of Absolute Knowledge, he wanders in the world, sometimes like a madman, sometimes like a child and at other times like a ghoul, having no other clothes on his person except the quarters, or sometimes wearing clothes, or perhaps skins at other times.[9]

The *siddhis* are spiritual milestones on the path of yoga. By attaining any such *siddhi,* the seeker gains faith in yoga and yoga practices, and this sustains him or her in the journey toward the goal.

Spiritual nourishment

Spiritual nourishment is vital for the seeker and a distinctive mark of spiritual advancement. Spiritual nourishment comes when the seeker is able to taste divine bliss in some form or other. The forerunner of the taste of bliss is a strong liking for holy company and the experience of contentment, peace, and joy. Contentment comes from tranquility of mind and desirelessness, and this brings peace. Peace is freedom from anxiety, fear, and the turbulence of the mind.

Spiritual practices have a taste that gives the seeker a joy of expansion. Nourishment becomes positive when the seeker tastes the bliss of the Self. The liberation of the soul, from Vedanta's point of view, is not merely freedom from pain but a taste of positive bliss. One who has tasted this bliss goes beyond all sorrow, fear, and anxiety. The *Katha Upanishad* says, "The wise man, having realized Atman as dwelling within impermanent bodies but Itself bodiless, vast, and all-pervading, does not grieve."[10]

Sri Ramakrishna describes joy of three kinds: *vishayananda*, that is, pleasure of the senses; *bhajanananda*, joy experienced by chanting the name of God and meditating on God; and the highest joy, *Brahmananda*, that is, the bliss of Brahman, or the Self:

> This is called bhajanananda, the bliss of devotees in the worship of God.... Through worship devotees receive the grace of God, and then His vision. Then they enjoy Brahmananda, the Bliss of Brahman.[11]

Having tasted the overpowering bliss of the Self, a seeker's mind does not want to return to the world of duality and multiplicity. Sri Ramakrishna describes that as you proceed toward the ocean, you feel the cool breeze of the ocean, hear the rumbling waves of the ocean, and finally you reach the ocean itself. By reaching the ocean of Brahman and bathing in its waves of bliss, you become ever satisfied and ever blessed. The seeker's spiritual advancement is measured in terms of the intensity of this taste of bliss.

Spiritual evolution from duty to absorption

The first stage of spiritual evolution is *karma-yoga*, where the seeker performs his or her spiritual practices with a sense of discipline and performs all actions, including prayer and meditation, with eyes open. *Karma-yoga* is practicing yoga in action. It is offering the results of karma to God. A seeker who is a worshipper of a personal God makes the offering to that personal God, and a non-dualist seeker offers all the results of karma to the flaming, luminous Self within.

In time, *karma-yoga* brings the seeker to the stage of *bhakti-yoga*, where the practices of yoga are done with love for the Divine. The feeling of discipline goes away and is replaced by the feeling of love. The seeker begins to get a taste of spiritual nourishment, the disciplines of renunciation and surrender to the Divine become easy, and there develops in the seeker an attachment to the Divine that culminates in pure love. *Bhakti-yoga* is keeping the mind focused on the Self.

Bhakti-yoga culminates in *raja-yoga*, where the seeker begins to feel absorption into the Divine. This absorption is meditation. Meditation has different depths and degrees: effortful, effortless, and spontaneous. *Raja-yoga* finally culminates in *jnana-yoga*, or the yoga of knowledge, in which state the seeker gets glimpses of the Divine and reaches the state of *samadhi*.

Karma-yoga collects the mind lost in the world of attachment and aversion. *Bhakti-yoga* keeps the mind devoted to the Divine. *Raja-yoga* keeps the devoted mind absorbed in the Divine. *Jnana-yoga* brings revelation of the Divine, where the mind communes with the Divine or becomes merged in it.

Rise and fall of the mind

Our mind experiences rises and falls. Even though the seat of the mind is between the eyebrows, the ordinary mind usually dwells at the lower three centers of consciousness (at the base of the spine, the organ of generation, and the region of the navel). Remaining at the lower three centers, the mind only broods over three things: eating, sleeping, and the pursuit of gross pleasures.

As described earlier, through spiritual practice, the mind begins to rise to the fourth center in the heart, the fifth in the throat, and the sixth between the eyebrows. Reaching the fourth center,

the seeker experiences glimpses of the Divine. The world, hith-
erto giving signals of eating, sleeping, and gross pleasures, now
appears unified. One experiences the light of Truth and gains
faith in the spiritual. Reaching the fifth center, one wants to hear
only about God—nothing else. Reaching the sixth, one becomes
silent and absorbed in the Divine.

But the mind again falls, because of the drags of old desires
and subtle impressions, known as *samskaras*. Spiritual advancement is measured in terms of the center to which the mind has
risen, its ability to dwell in that region for a longer and longer period of time, and by observing whether this rising of the mind
happens consciously.

Transformation of ego

Ego is the root cause of all the problems of life. It denies the
existence of others and creates spiritual blindness. At the social
level, it brings maladjustment and creates more enemies than
friends; at the psychological level, it creates a kind of fever, anxiety, and depression; in spiritual life, it creates countless road-
blocks of doubt, denial, hopelessness, and despair. But the ego is
both the troublemaker and the troubleshooter.

Ego is the personality. It creates diversity and novelty and
projects the world of imagination and fantasy by blocking the
light of reality that reveals the oneness of existence. Ego first creates attachment, then brings a sense of duty, then brings agony,
and thereafter looks for a solution. It is the primary roadblock to
harmonious human relations and social adjustment necessary for
peace of mind. In brief, the ego brings swelling of the head and
shrinking of the heart.

The ego cannot be denied, crushed, or ignored. It can only be
transformed and matured. Sri Ramakrishna says:

> The "ego of Devotion," the "ego of Knowledge," and the "ego
> of a child" do not harm the devotee.... The bhakta feels, "O God,

Thou art the Lord and I am Thy devotee." This "I" is the "ego of bhakti." Why does such a lover of God retain the "ego of Devotion"? There is a reason. The ego cannot be got rid of; so let the rascal remain as the servant of God, the devotee of God.[12]

As discussed previously, the ego has three faces in keeping with the three *gunas*. The *tamasika* or infantile ego takes delight in being nothing, in crying, cringing, and cursing. It does not have any sense of value. It lives on charity and the favors of others. The *rajasika* or immature ego takes delight in being somebody important. It takes pride in worldly accomplishment and power. Its credo is "I am the lord of all; I enjoy; I am prosperous, mighty and happy; I am rich; I am of high birth. Who else is equal to me?"[13] The watchword of the *sattvika* or mature ego is "I am honest and good; I have renounced everything for the sake of God; I am holy; I sacrifice myself for the good of all beings." The *sattvika* ego takes delight in spiritual wealth. It creates attachment to knowledge and happiness.

In other words, examine the ego: if it is *tamasika*, put it to work. It needs self-assertion and self-development by becoming active, efficient, and accomplished. If it is *rajasika*, the ego needs to be reduced. Lessen the ego by being spiritually active, humble, and self-controlled. If it is *sattvika*, the ego must surrender itself to the Divine.

Spiritual progress is measured by observing the transformation of the ego from *tamasika* to the *sattvika* stage and changes in the *guna* composition. The ideal condition is when *tamas* and *rajas* are subordinated to *sattva guna*.

Dreams

Dreams indicate the dreamer's inner nature. From a strictly spiritual point of view, a dream is a dream and not a reality. Vedanta emphasizes the importance of the wakeful state and the seeker's spiritual struggles in that state.

A seeker is considered progressing when even in a dream the spiritual struggles continue, when in a dream he or she also makes the utmost effort to combat the old tendencies and meditate on the Divine. Such signs indicate that the seeker's subconscious is being transformed and that spirituality has struck a deep root in the mind.

Mastery of the spiritual virtues

Mastery over the positive spiritual virtues is a sure sign of spiritual progress. These virtues are dispassion, discrimination, self-control, renunciation, devotion, and knowledge. But each of these virtues has its counterpart.

Discrimination becomes useless without dispassion; dispassion, which is distaste for worldly enjoyment, is false without devotion. A seeker may dislike worldly enjoyment, but then the question arises: What is his or her source of enjoyment? Life must have enjoyment. The seeker's passionlessness for worldly enjoyment must be balanced by a passion for God; otherwise, it may be considered depression.

Self-control, which is mastery over the mind and senses, becomes repressive when not practiced for the sake of Self-knowledge. Renunciation without the spirit of service is an escape, which is never spiritual. Knowledge of the Self in meditation is incomplete unless that knowledge is translated in the form of action. The depth of devotion, when not matched by an equal depth of dispassion, is a cheap sentiment. Self-knowledge without the spirit of self-dedication to the welfare of all beings is sterile.

By taking into account each positive virtue and its counterpart, seekers on the path of yoga can ascertain the extent of their spiritual progress.

Longing for the Divine

Longing for the Divine is a sure mark of spiritual progress. As the seeker advances along the spiritual path, his or her longing for Self-knowledge or God-vision begins to increase. This long-ing takes over the whole mind of the seeker, making him or her intensely restless for the goal. As Sri Ramakrishna says:

> Longing is like the rosy dawn. After the dawn out comes the sun. Longing is followed by the vision of God....

> There are certain signs of God-realization. A man who longs for God is not far from attaining Him. What are the outer in-dications of such longing? They are discrimination, dispas-sion, compassion for living beings, serving holy men, loving their company, chanting God's name and glories, telling the truth, and the like. When you see those signs in an aspirant, you can rightly say that for him the vision of God is not far to seek....

> At the approach of dawn the eastern horizon becomes red. Then one knows it will soon be sunrise. Likewise, if you see a person restless for God, you can be pretty certain that he hasn't long to wait for His vision.[14]

Spiritual longing, in order to be authentic, must be backed up by discrimination, dispassion, and self-control. The seeker's in-tensity of longing also makes these practices intense. Without such longing, the seeker's practices become nominal and he or she fails to make significant progress.

The desire for holy company is an important aspect of long-ing for the Divine. A person on the spiritual path feels drawn to the company of holy persons who have renounced everything for God and attained God-realization. Only by meeting such holy persons and associating with them does a seeker gain faith in God and in the reality of the spiritual goal. One can never attain complete faith in God simply by the study of sacred texts, philo-sophical reasoning, and spiritual practice. One must have the company of a realized soul. Sri Ramakrishna says:

> The constant company of holy men is necessary. They intro-duce one to God.[15]

Repeat God's name and sing His glories, and now and then visit God's devotees and holy men. The mind cannot dwell on God if it is immersed day and night in worldliness, in worldly duties and responsibilities; it is most necessary to go into solitude now and then and think of God.[16]

The Bhagavad Gita tells us:

Learn it by prostration, by inquiry, and by [personal] service. The wise, who have seen the Truth, will teach you that Knowledge.[17]

By associating with holy persons, a spiritual seeker is able to judge where he or she stands on the spiritual path. This is not possible by self-analysis alone. The seeker's intensity of longing for the Divine is reflected in the seeker's increased desire for holy company and serving the holy.

11

Vital Spiritual Questions and Their Answers

In order to reach the goal of the spiritual quest, the Bhagavad Gita maintains that the spiritual seeker must strive by "right means."[1] But what is the meaning of *right means?* The yogi is asked to be "temperate in his food and recreation, temperate in his exertion at work, temperate in sleep and waking," and for one who is temperate, "yoga puts an end to all sorrows."[2] Are there any specific guidelines in this regard?

Explaining the meaning of yoga and its practice, the *Katha Upanishad* says, "This, the firm control of the senses, is what is called yoga. One must then be vigilant; for yoga can be both beneficial and injurious."[3] *Beneficial and injurious* may mean that yoga can be both acquired and lost. The question is raised as to how yoga can be both beneficial and injurious, or why yoga can be both acquired and lost?

Further, the Bhagavad Gita says, "For a sage who wants to attain yoga, action is said to be the means; but when he has attained yoga, serenity is said to be the means."[4]

Withdrawal from all activities is being recommended for one, while selfless action for self-purification is being recommended for another. How should one know whether one has attained yoga or not?

The spiritual seeker is often troubled by questions and doubts along the journey and looks for straightforward answers. The following is an attempt to provide some answers, as given by the sacred texts and traditions of Vedanta and Yoga.

Does God listen to my prayer?

Spiritual seekers are often assailed by doubts about whether their prayers reach God and whether God listens to their prayers. Regarding this, Sri Ramakrishna says:

One must be restless for God. If a son clamours persistently for his share of the property, his parents consult with each other and give it to him even though he is a minor. God will certainly listen to your prayers if you feel restless for Him. He has begotten us, surely we can claim our inheritance from Him. He is our own Father, our own Mother. We can force our demand on Him. We can say to Him, "Reveal Thyself to me or I shall cut my throat with a knife!" ...

I used to pray to [the Divine Mother] in this way: "O Mother! O Blissful One! Reveal Thyself to me. Thou must!" Again, I would say to Her: "O Lord of the lowly! O Lord of the universe! Surely I am not outside Thy universe. I am bereft of knowledge. I am without discipline. I have no devotion. I know nothing. Thou must be gracious and reveal Thyself to me."[5]

Again, in another context, Sri Ramakrishna assures the devotees about the efficacy of prayer:

Hazra: Does God listen to our prayer for bhakti [devotion]?

Master: Surely. I can assure you of that a hundred times. But the prayer must be genuine and earnest. Do worldly-minded people weep for God as they do for wife and children? At Kamarpukur the wife of a certain man fell ill. The man thought she would not recover; he began to tremble and was about to faint. Who feels that way for God?[6]

You will feel restless for God when your heart becomes pure and your mind free from attachment to the things of the world. Then alone will your prayer reach God. A telegraph wire cannot carry messages if it has a break or some other defect.[7]

Pundit Shashadar, a renowned Hindu preacher of the time, asked Sri Ramakrishna, "Does God listen to our prayers?" Sri Ramakrishna answered:

God is the Kalpataru, the Wish-fulfilling Tree. You will certainly get whatever you ask of Him. But you must pray standing near the Kalpataru. Only then will your prayer be fulfilled. But you must remember another thing. God knows our inner feeling. A man gets the fulfillment of the desire he cherishes while practicing sadhana. As one thinks, so one receives.[8]

The question is addressed in an exchange between Holy Mother Sarada Devi and a devotee:

Devotee: Mother, if I pray to the Master silently, will he listen? And should I say anything to the Master without letting you know first?

Mother grew somewhat agitated on hearing this and said, "If he be true, certainly he will hear you."

Devotee: It is said that one realizes God by praying to Him sincerely for two or three days. I have been praying for such a long time, but why do I not get any realization?

Mother: Everything will come in time, my child. The words of Sri Ramakrishna ... can never be in vain. Be devoted to him and take shelter at his feet. It is enough to remember that there is some One, call Him father or mother, who is always protecting you.

Lay the burden of your mind before Sri Ramakrishna. Tell him your sorrows with your tears. You will find that he will fill your hands with the desired objects.

[Sri Ramakrishna] used to say, "One who remembers me never suffers from want of food or from physical privations."... By remembering him one gets rid of all sufferings.[9]

In the *Uddhava Gita,* Sri Krishna says:

With a view to purify Myself by the dust of his feet, I always follow the sage who cares for nothing, is calm, bears enmity to none, and is even-minded.[10]

In the Bhagavad Gita, Sri Krishna assures spiritual seekers with his promise:

Those persons who worship Me, meditating on their identity with Me and ever devoted to Me—to them I carry what they lack and for them I preserve what they already have.

[T]here is no destruction for him either in this world or the next: no evil, My son, befalls a man who does good.

The man who has fallen away from yoga goes to the worlds of the righteous. Having lived there for unnumbered years, he is reborn in the home of the pure and the prosperous.

Or, he is born in a family of yogis rich in wisdom. Verily, such birth is hard to gain in this world.

Even the most sinful man, if he worships Me with unswerving devotion, must be regarded as righteous; for he has formed the right resolution.

He soon becomes righteous and attains eternal peace. Proclaim it boldly... that My devotee never perishes.

Whoever offers Me, with devotion, a leaf, a flower, a fruit, or water—that I accept, the pious offering of the pure heart.[11]

In regard to prayer, Christ says:

But thou, when thou prayest, enter into thy closet, and when thou hast shut thy door, pray to thy Father which is in secret; and thy Father which seeth in secret shall reward thee openly. (Matt. 6:6)

Prayer is the outpouring of the soul. It is making a direct appeal to God. It is the last refuge of a spiritual seeker when all other means of attaining God have failed. Prayer does not have any definite language. It can be verbal, semi-verbal, or silent. Sincere prayer is always answered. This is the assurance of the prophets, saints, and scriptures of different traditions.

For receiving an answer to prayer a seeker is required to be wholehearted, true in thought, word, and deed, and intensely restless for an answer. One must throw oneself completely at the mercy of God. The cry of a sincere soul is never ignored by God, since all souls are God's created beings. Spiritual illumination, which alone puts an end to all sufferings of life, is not the result of human effort. Spiritual illumination is the gift of God that comes as divine grace. Only sincere prayer makes divine intervention possible.

What is the meaning of "mantra"?

The mantra is a sacred word imparted by the teacher to a disciple. Repetition of a mantra purifies the mind and leads to concentration and meditation. The mantra has two powers: saving and transforming. Repetition of a mantra saves a seeker from the calamities of life. It counters the evil results of past karma. Holy Mother Sri Sarada Devi says:

> One must experience the effect of past action. None can escape it. But *japa* [repetition of a mantra] minimizes its intensity. For example, a man who, as a result of his past karma, is destined to lose his leg, may instead suffer from the prick of a thorn in his foot.[12]

The other power is transforming power. Repetition of a mantra transforms the consciousness of the seeker and leads to illumination. The tradition of Tantra claims that constant repetition of a mantra itself is enough for illumination. The power of a mantra is unfailing. Holy Mother says, "The mind will be steadied of itself if aspirants repeat God's name fifteen or twenty thousand times a day. I myself have experienced it."[13]

According to *Siva Sutra,* the mantra is not the letters constituting it. The mind has to dwell on its meaning, to discriminate between the real and the unreal in the light of knowledge and become united with the truth embodied in the mantra. The process of grasping the meaning of the mantra and soaking oneself in its consciousness is the real *japa,* or *mantra-sadhana.*[14]

According to *Parasurama Kalpasutra,* the power of the mantra is inconceivable and limitless.[15] This power comes from three sources: first, the mantra is a living form of the deity; second, it is charged with the power of austerity of the seer who envisioned the mantra; third, the guru from whom the mantra is received imparts to it his or her own power and transmits that power to the disciple. When one repeats the mantra in "due order," one automatically invokes the power of the deity, the power of the seer of the mantra, and the power of the guru—all combining to form a dynamo of power. *Due order* implies that the mantra has been received from one authorized to give it and that it is repeated in the right spirit and form.

The mantra must be received from a guru and not just picked up by oneself.[16] The guru must be one who has the authority to initiate another into the mantra. The guru must belong to the line of gurus, each of whom in the past has empowered the mantra with purity and austerity. Only then can the power and purity of all the gurus in the tradition be active in the mantra.

What is mantra siddhi?

A potent mantra imparted by an illumined teacher, when repeated with devotion and faith, becomes awakened. Repetition constitutes feeding the mantra. When not fed, due to negligence or forgetfulness on the part of the seeker, the mantra eats up the reserves of spiritual merit previously acquired by the seeker. But when fed and adored properly, repetition of the mantra purifies the body and mind. As Holy Mother Sri Sarada Devi says:

> As wind removes the cloud, so the name of God destroys the cloud of worldliness.... Repeating the name of God once with the mind controlled is equivalent to a million repetitions with the mind away from God. You may repeat the name for the whole day, but if the mind is elsewhere, that does not produce much result. The repetition must be accompanied by concentration. Then alone one gets the grace of God.[17]

Is mechanical repetition of the mantra of any use?

Holy Mother assures the seeker of the effectiveness of *japa*:

> A disciple asked the [Holy] Mother if the mere repetition of the holy word taught by a qualified guru helped the aspirant, if he did not possess intense devotion. "Whether you jump into water or are pushed into it," she replied, "your cloth will be soaked, will it not?"[18]

How much time should I spend in *japa*, meditation, worship, and scriptural studies?

Regarding the length of time to be devoted to meditation, Swami Vidyaranya, in his *Jivan-Mukti-Viveka*, gives the following guidelines:

> The beginner should follow the right course of yoga thus: he should fill two parts of his mind with objects of enjoyment, one part by the study of the scriptures, and one part by attending on his preceptor.
>
> When he has progressed to some extent, then he should fill one part of his mind with objects of enjoyment, one part by reflecting on the scriptures, and the remaining two parts by attending upon the preceptor.

When quite advanced, he should fill half of his mind by study of scriptures and practice of renunciation, and the remaining half by meditation and worshiping his teacher.[19]

The *Amritanda-Upanishad* says:

A Yogi should always avoid fear, anger, laziness, too much sleep or waking and too much food and fasting. If the above rules be well strictly practised each day, spiritual wisdom will arise of itself in three months without doubt. In four months, he sees the Devas; in five months, he knows (or becomes) Brahmanishta [dedicated to Brahman]; and truly in six months, he attains Kaivalya [perfection of aloneness] at will. There is no doubt.[20]

Swami Brahmananda, Sri Ramakrishna's eminent direct disciple, says the following:

Devote as much time as possible to japam and meditation and to worship and study. Those who want to lead a purely contemplative life should spend at least sixteen hours a day in japam and meditation. As you continue your practice, you will be able to increase the time. The more the mind is turned inward, the more joy you will get. Once you get joy in meditation, it will be hard to discontinue it. Then you will no longer have to ask how long you should meditate. Your mind will tell you. Before you reach this stage, try to spend two-thirds of the day in japam and meditation, and the rest of the time in study of the scriptures and self-introspection. It is not enough to practice meditation closing the eyes for an hour. One should examine the mind and eliminate its subtle cravings for the world. Then when the mind becomes calm, one can get deep meditation. The goal of spiritual practices is to calm the mind. If your mind is not tranquil and if you do not get joy within, remember, you are not on the right track.[21]

Sometimes the mind does not want to practice meditation. Should I force myself to meditate, or occupy myself with *japa* or study of the scriptures?

Swami Brahmananda answers:

It is the nature of the mind to rebel against effort and to always seek comforts. If you want to achieve something you will have to work hard. In the preliminary stage in order to cultivate a strong habit, you must force your mind to meditate. If you find it difficult to sit for long hours, lie down on your bed and practice japam. If you feel sleepy, walk and repeat the mantram. In this way the habit will be formed. Never give up your sadhana. You must wage war against the mind. To bring the mind under control is the goal of spiritual disciplines.[22]

How much time should I devote to sleep?

Regarding this, Swami Brahmananda says:

Ordinarily for a healthy person four hours' sleep is quite sufficient. Some may need one or two hours more. To sleep more than five hours is a disease. Too much sleep does not give the body rest. On the contrary, it does harm to the body. It is not good for an aspirant to waste time in sleep. You are young. This is the best time to train the mind. Later you will get plenty of time to sleep. So often when a person is asked to practice sadhana, he immediately raises a number of lame excuses. He says that his body will not be able to bear such strain, that he needs more rest, and so on. Such an insincere person seeks only rest and comfort without doing anything. If one practices japam and meditation sincerely, one's senses and nerves move in a very rhythmic way, and as a result, four hours' sleep is sufficient. Generally most people lead irregular lives and their bodies and minds are so tired they do not get rest even after eight or ten hours' sleep. Try to regulate your life like a clock. Regulation will keep the body and mind fresh.[23]

Regarding rules for sleep for a spiritual seeker, the *Manu-Smriti* observes:

If the sun should rise or set while he is still sleeping, either intentionally or unintentionally, he should fast during the day, reciting (the Savitri). If during one's sleep the sun has set, and if during one's sleep the sun has risen—if he does not perform the Expiatory Rite, he becomes tainted by grievous sin.[24]

According to the commentary on this verse:

He who becomes tainted by the setting of the sun—similarly who becomes tainted by the rising of the sun—and he does not perform the expiatory rite prescribed above, then he becomes tainted by *grievous*—not minor—*sin.* "Sin" is the name of that unseen force which leads one to suffer pain in the form of living in hell and so forth.[25]

What rules regarding food should I observe? Should I eat whatever I am given or should I discriminate?

Regarding this, Swami Brahmananda says:

During sadhana it is better to have a little discrimination about food. Some kinds of food increase sleepiness and should be avoided. It is not good to eat too many sweets, sour pickles, or urad lentils. These foods increase tamas in the body, which means more laziness and more sleep. It is almost impossible for a man of tamasic nature to practice sadhana. Eat that food which is easily digestible. Never fill your stomach more than two-thirds with food. This will increase your strength and energy.[26]

Regarding food and sleep, the Bhagavad Gita says, "Yoga is not for him who eats too much nor for him who eats too little. It is not for him, O Arjuna, who sleeps too much nor for him who sleeps too little."[27]

According to the books on yoga, a yogi should fill half of the stomach with food, one quarter with water, and leave one quarter empty for the movement of air. According to another view, five things are indispensable for success in meditation: practice of silence, a light diet of milk and fruits, living in solitude, personal contact with the teacher, and a cool place. Concentration and meditation should be practiced with an empty stomach, empty bladder, and an empty colon, and a salt-free diet is immensely helpful in that regard.

About vegetarianism, Swami Saradananda says:

You have asked me whether vegetarianism is absolutely necessary for leading a spiritual life. My answer is that no hard and fast rule can be made with regard to food. Can we live without doing harm to some form of life? Do you think plants and vegetables have no life? Our scriptures say they have; science has proven it. If you preserve the strength and vigor of your body and mind while living on vegetarian food, you are at liberty to do so. But if, while foregoing fish and meat, your health deteriorates, you must give up such ideas and take a more moderate stand. As a general rule, when the body becomes weak, the mind is weakened also. A weak mind is unfit for meditation. When a man with such a mind tries to meditate, his mind runs away. It is only a strong person with sufficient will power who can concentrate and fix his mind on God. Therefore, you must not do anything that will impair your spiritual life. Whatever you eat, make it an offering to the Lord. You are to think that God resides in the body in the form of fire and that the food you eat is given as an oblation to the fire.... It is for this reason that monks in India make a firm resolve not to take meals without reciting the following verse from the Gita: "Brahman is the ritual, Brahman is the offering, Brahman is he who offers to the fire that is Brahman. If a mind sees Brahman in every action, he will find Brahman."[28]

The object of food is to build a strong body and a fine intellect. Unless the body and the mind are pure it is not possible
to do spiritual practices. It is the food offered to God that
builds a pure body and mind.[29]

Regarding the necessity of nourishing food, Swami
Vivekananda recalls the following incident:

One day a young man brought to me in the house of Mohini
Babu at Dacca, a photograph and said, "Sir, please tell me
who he is. Is he an Avatara?" I told him gently many times that
I knew nothing of it. When even on my telling him three or four
times the boy did not cease from his persistent questioning,
I was constrained to say at last: "My boy, henceforward take
a little nutritious food and then your brain will develop. Without
nourishing food, I see your brain has dried up." At these words
the young man may have been much displeased. But what
could I do? Unless I spoke like this to the boys, they would
turn into madcaps by degrees.[30]

Purity of food also includes the purity of mental food, that is,
whatever a person enjoys through the five organs of perception—
sight, sound, touch, taste, and smell. The essence of the purity
of mental food is chastity in thought, word, and deed under all
circumstances.

What are the rules regarding my clothing?

Clothing made out of natural products, such as cotton or
wool, is said to be conducive to the practice of meditation and
concentration. Further, the clothes worn by the seeker should be
new and not used by anyone before. They should be clean, simple, and unostentatious. Unostentatious dress deflects the gaze of
the worldly minded. Regarding this question of clothing, Swami
Brahmananda says:

You should have enough clothing to protect yourself from heat
and cold. As you are a monk, it is not good for you to collect

a lot of clothing and carry it in a bundle. You should not accept anything extra, even if somebody offers it to you. On the other hand, your goal is God-realization and not hardship. An aspirant cannot concentrate on God if he suffers from too much heat or cold. Wear enough clothing to maintain your good health. Procuring many things for enjoyment is luxury, which is extremely dangerous for monastic life. It is terrible to beg for luxurious things from people.[31]

What is the best season for spiritual practices?

According to Swami Saradananda:

The rainy season is not suited to them [spiritual practices]. One gets drowsy when one tries to meditate. We experienced this. In that season the mind becomes more restless. Winter is best suited for meditation.[32]

What is the meaning of "shrine in the heart"?

Seekers are often asked to meditate and concentrate in the shrine of the heart, where God dwells as the inmost Self. Shankaracharya explains the meaning of this practice:

He who, renouncing all activities, worships in the sacred and stainless shrine of Atman, which is independent of time, place, and distance; which is present everywhere; which is the destroyer of heat and cold, and the other opposites; and which is the giver of eternal happiness, becomes all-knowing and all-pervading and attains, hereafter, Immortality.[33]

According to a commentary on this verse:

The word *shrine* in the text also means a holy place (*tirtha*). The allusion is to the pilgrimage of pious devotees to a holy place. There are certain disadvantages associated with holy places. As they may be situated at a great distance, pilgrimage may entail physical labour and suffering. The merit of a pilgrimage may be slight because of the inauspiciousness of the time. The comfort of the pilgrims may be disturbed by the weather. Robbers, thieves, or unscrupulous priests often give them trouble. Further, the merit accruing from a pilgrimage is not everlasting. But the worshipper in the sacred shrine of Atman is free from all these disadvantages and obstacles. Communion with Atman bestows upon the soul Immortality and Eternal Bliss.

The *Mahabharata* describes Atman as the real sacred river, bathing in which the soul becomes free of impurities:

"The river of Atman is filled with the water of self-control; truth is its current, righteous conduct its banks, and compassion its waves. O son of Pandu, bathe in its sacred water; ordinary water does not purify the inmost soul."

By worshipping a holy man who worships in the sacred shrine of Atman, the seeker obtains the result of pilgrimage:

"A visit to holy men bestows merit, because they may be regarded as moving holy places. The Lord, dwelling in their hearts, renders holy the place where they live.

"A river filled with sacred water is no doubt sacred; an image of stone or clay is no doubt a deity. After worshipping them a long time, the aspirant becomes pure. But by a mere visit to a holy man one attains purity."

Communion with Brahman is the most efficacious form of worship: "By virtue of even a moment's serenity, attained through the knowledge of the identity of Atman and Brahman, the seeker attains the merit that one may obtain by bathing in the waters of all the holy rivers, by giving away the entire world in an act of charity, by performing a thousand sacrifices, by worshipping the three hundred and thirty millions of gods, and by rescuing, through after-death rites, one's ancestors from the suffering of the nether world.

"By the very birth of a man whose mind is absorbed in the Supreme Brahman—the immeasurable Ocean of Existence-Knowledge-Bliss Absolute—his family becomes sinless, his mother blessed, and the earth sacred."[34]

How can I attain liberation?

Shankaracharya replies to this question:

Let people quote the scriptures and sacrifice to the gods, let them perform rituals and worship the deities, but there is no liberation without the realization of one's identity with the Atman, no, not even in the lifetime of a hundred Brahmās put together. [That is, an indefinite length of time. One day of Brahmā (the Creator) is 432 million years.][35]

Neither by Yoga [may mean *hatha yoga,* which strengthens the body], nor by Sankhya, nor by work [work for material ends, such as getting to heaven and so forth, is meant], nor by learning, but by the realization of one's identity with Brahman is liberation possible, and by no other means. [None of these, if practiced mechanically, will bring on the highest knowledge, the absolute identity of the Jiva and Brahman, which alone, according to Advaita Vedanta, is the supreme way to liberation.][36]

What are the marks of Self-knowledge?

According to Shankaracharya, the marks are the following:

The *yogin* who has attained perfection and is liberated-in-life gets this as result—he enjoys eternal Bliss in his mind, internally as well as externally.

The result of dispassion is knowledge, that of knowledge is withdrawal from sense-pleasures, which leads to the experience of the Bliss of the Self, whence follows Peace.

If there is an absence of the succeeding stages, the preceding ones are futile. (When the series is perfect) the cessation of the objective world, extreme satisfaction, and matchless bliss follow as a matter of course.

Being unruffled by earthly troubles is the result in question of knowledge. How can a man who did various loathsome deeds during the state of delusion, commit the same afterwards, possessed of discrimination?

The result of knowledge should be the turning away from unreal things, while attachment to these is the result of ignorance. This is observed in the case of one who knows a mirage and things of that sort, and one who does not. Otherwise, what other tangible result do the knowers of Brahman obtain?

If the heart's knot of ignorance is totally destroyed, what natural cause can there be for inducing such a man to selfish action—the man who is averse to sense-pleasures?

When the sense-objects excite no more desire, then is the culmination of dispassion. The extreme perfection of knowledge is the absence of any impulsion of the egoistic idea. And the limit of self-withdrawal is reached when the mind-functions that have been merged, appear no more.[37]

What is spiritual vibration?

"Our thoughts, feelings, and wills are like waves in the mind,"[38] and these waves are called vibrations. Different waves vibrate at different rates.

The Upanishads tell us that there are three rates of vibration, modes, corresponding to three colours—white, red, and black. Black stands for *Tamas* or dull forces; Red for *Rajas,* the tense forces of desire and greed; White indicates *Sattva,* the harmonious forces of purity…. These ideas are strange to Western minds, but they were familiar to Plato….

In his "Republic" he speaks of three active principles which he calls Epithumia, Thumos, and Logistikon, corresponding to

Tamas, Rajas, and Sattva. The first force, Epithumia, is, he says, a multiplicity of blind appetites or desires which dominate the votaries of sensuous enjoyments, and whose chief aim is the gratification of animal appetites. Thumos ... dominates the man of action who works with frenzied zeal for distinction or worldly position and power; grasping and greedy ... [and] filled with restless unhappiness. Logistikon, like Sattva, represents the rational elements characterising the philosopher and sage, such as detachment, moderation, purity and harmony.

These three types of forces are at work within us at all times. When we say that a person has too much tamas we mean that the dull, dark forces overshadow, for the time being, the other two types. When a person is ruled by passion and desire we say that Rajas is predominant. If his life is peaceful and harmonious, if he seems to have detached himself from worldly desires, we say that Sattva rules. These are the three gunas.[39]

Vibrations can be worldly or spiritual. "In the life of Sri Ramakrishna we find how he was unable to drink a cup of water brought to him by an apparently decent-looking man who, it was later discovered, was leading an impure life. Swami Vivekananda relates how, when his own vibrations were bad, the Master could not take food from his hands.... Vibrations can be changed, the impure can become pure."[40] Worldly vibrations can be overcome by consciously cultivating spiritual thoughts and habits. Swami Vivekananda said:

Every part of the body can be filled with prana, the vital force; and when you are able to do that, you can control the whole body. All the sickness and misery felt in the body will be perfectly controlled. Not only so, but you will be able to control another's body. Everything is infectious in this world—good or bad. If your body is in a certain state of tension, it will have a tendency to produce the same tension in others. If you are strong and healthy, those who live near you will also have a tendency to become strong and healthy; but if you are sick and weak, those around you will have a tendency to become the same. In the case of one man's trying to heal another, the first step is simply to transfer his own health to the other. This is a primitive way of healing. Consciously or unconsciously, health can be transmitted....

The pure-souled man who has controlled his prana has the power to bring it into a certain state of vibration which can be conveyed to others, arousing in them a similar vibration. You see that in everyday actions. I am talking to you. What am I trying to do? I am, in reality, bringing my mind to a certain state of vibration, and the more I succeed in bringing it to that state, the more you will be affected by what I say....

The world-movers, endowed with gigantic will-power, can bring their prana into a high state of vibration; and it is so great and powerful that it affects others in a moment, and thousands are drawn towards them, and half the world think as they do. The great prophets of the world had the most wonderful control of their prana, which gave them tremendous will-power; they had brought their prana to the highest state of vibration, and this is what gave them power to sway the world.[41]

What is the role of a spiritual teacher?

Tantra and Vedanta contend that there is no illumination without a spiritual teacher, or guru. There are a hundred different paths leading to the Divine, just as there are a hundred different natures in humanity. It is not possible for an individual seeker to know what is best for himself or herself. The guru chooses the seeker's path according to the seeker's natural abilities and spiritual development.

There are numerous potholes on the spiritual quest and numberless delusions and temptations that stand in the way. It is the guru who protects and guides the seeker. Swami Vivekananda says, "The guru is the means of realization. There is no knowledge without a teacher.'"[42]

> The guru is the conveyance through which the spiritual influence is brought to you. Anyone can teach, but the spirit is transmitted only by the guru to the sishya, the disciple, and that will fructify. The relation between sishyas is that of brotherhood, and this is actually accepted by law in India. The guru passes the thought-power, the mantra, that he has received from those before him; and nothing can be done without a guru—in fact great danger ensues. Usually without a guru these yoga practices lead to lust; but with one this seldom happens. Each Ishta has a mantra. The Ishta is the ideal peculiar to the particular worshipper; the mantra is the external word to express it. Constant repetition of the word helps to fix the ideal firmly in the mind. This method of worship prevails among religious devotees all over India.[43]

The *Kularnava Tantra* says, "As human, the guru is seen by the sinner; as divine by the meritful."[44] The ignorant see only the human exterior and look upon the guru as a mere human being. But a true seeker looks upon the teacher as the Supreme Guru, God, who, assuming a human disguise, has come to bless the seeker.

The *Parasurama Kalpa Sutra* asks for absolute loyalty to one guru, because the guru is the spiritual mother or father of the disciple.[45] The guru's obligation to the disciple continues from birth to birth, until the disciple attains illumination. The spiritual progress of spiritual seekers depends upon their faithfulness to the guru, who constantly accompanies them in their path in the form of "guru-power." When one seeks guidance from a second guru, one loses the protective power of the original guru and becomes vulnerable to conflicting influences.

The spiritual life of a seeker is like a plant that, in order to grow, must remain rooted in one soil. Changing it from one soil to another can destroy it.

How should I regard my teacher, father, mother, and others?

The ancient Hindu lawgiver Manu says:

The preceptor, the father, the mother and the elder brother should not be treated with disrespect, especially by a Brahmana—even though he be distressed [by them]. The preceptor is the embodiment of Brahman; the father is the embodiment of Prajapati [the creator]; the Mother is the embodiment of the earth; and one's own brother is the embodiment of the self. The trouble that the parents undergo in the birth of children—for that there can be no compensation even in a hundred years. He should always do what is pleasing to those two and to the preceptor; on these three being satisfied, all austerity becomes completed. The service of these three is declared to be the highest austerity; until permitted by them, one should not perform any other meritorious act....

The householder who fails not towards these three would win the three regions, and rejoice in heaven, radiant in body, like a God. He acquires this region by devotion to his Mother, the middle region by devotion to his Father, and the region of Brahman by serving his Preceptor. All the duties have been honoured by him who has honoured these three; and all acts remain fruitless for him who does not honour them. So long as these three live, he should not do anything else; he should always render service unto them, rejoicing in what is pleasing and beneficial to them.... The Brahmana who, till the dissolution of his body, serves his teacher, goes forthwith to the eternal abode of Brahman.[46]

Are there rules for the teacher as well as the taught?

According to Manu:

One should not instruct anyone unless he has asked, and not anyone who asks in an improper manner. Even though knowing [the truth], the wise man should behave among men as if ignorant. He who instructs in an unlawful manner and he who asks in an unlawful manner—of those two, one or the other either dies [untimely] or incurs the ill will [of the people]. Learning should not be sown where there is neither religion nor profit, nor at least suitable obedience, just as good seed (should not be sown) on salt soil.[47]

What is the meaning of initiation?

Initiation into a sacred mantra by the guru is a vital spiritual necessity. When seekers first inquire about the spiritual quest, they struggle by themselves for a while, then become initiated into a sacred path by a guru, and attain their spiritual birth. They now belong to the lineage and spiritual family of their guru, and their connection with the guru is eternal. According to *Parasurama Kalpasutra,* when the guru initiates the disciple, part of the guru enters into the being of the disciple and links the consciousness of the disciple with the guru. Eventually the disciple becomes one in spirit and mind with the guru.[48]

There is a view that the sins of the disciple visit the guru. Holy Mother Sarada Devi confirms this view:

> The guru imparts spiritual power to the disciple through the mystic syllable at the time of the initiation. The spiritual powers flow from the Guru to the disciple or vice versa. That is why after initiation of a disciple one gets ill, for one has to take the sins of the disciple. That is why Rakhal (Swami Brahmananda) is reluctant to initiate people. He says that immediately after initiating people he gets ill. But if the disciple is good, the Guru is benefited thereby. Some people get a sudden spiritual awakening immediately after initiation, but that depends upon one's samskaras (past tendencies).[49]

Swami Vivekananda says:

> To play the role of a spiritual teacher is a very difficult thing. One has to take on oneself the sins of others. There is every

chance of a fall in a less advanced man. If merely physical pain ensues, then he should consider himself fortunate.[50]

What is the main obstacle in the spiritual path?

The sacred texts of Yoga and Vedanta mention various obstacles that beset the path of yoga, such as inertia, inability to concentrate, distractions of sense pleasure, taste of bliss, attachment, aversion, delusion, and desire. But all these various obstacles are many ramifications of one main obstacle, which Sri Ramakrishna indicates as "lust and greed." In *The Gospel of Sri Ramakrishna*, the Master repeatedly warns spiritual seekers about this obstacle.

> The obstacle to yoga is "woman and gold" [lust and greed].* Yoga is possible when the mind becomes pure. The seat of the mind is between the eyebrows; but its look is fixed on the navel and the organs of generation and evacuation, that is to say, on "woman and gold." But through spiritual discipline the same mind looks upward.[51]

> If you want to realize God, then you must cultivate intense dispassion. You must renounce immediately what you feel to be standing in your way. You should not put it off till the future. "Woman and gold" is the obstruction. The mind must be withdrawn from it.[52]

> Some are born with the characteristic of a yogi; but they too should be careful. It is "woman and gold" alone that is the obstacle; it makes them deviate from the path of yoga and drags them into worldliness.[53]

> If the mind is free from "woman and gold," then what else can obstruct a man? He enjoys then only the Bliss of Brahman.[54]

---

*"The term 'woman and gold' ... occurs again and again in the teachings of Sri Ramakrishna to designate the chief impediments to spiritual progress. This favourite expression of the Master, 'kaminikanchan,' has often been misconstrued. *By it he meant only 'lust and greed,'* the baneful influence of

It is said that mastery over the pallet and sex instinct is the essence of all self-control and the highest of austerities. Without this mastery, Self-knowledge for the spiritual seeker is an empty dream.

What is the meaning of self-control?

Regarding this question, Manu says:

The wise man should put forth an effort to restrain his organs roaming among alluring objects; just as the driver restrains the horses. Those eleven organs which the ancient sages have named, I shall now fully describe in due order. [They are] the ear, the skin, the eyes, the tongue and the nose as the fifth; the anus, the generative organ, the hands and the feet, and speech described as the tenth. Of these, the five beginning with the ear in due order they call "organs of sensation," and five of these beginning with the anus, "organs of action." The mind is to be regarded as the eleventh, which, by its own quality, is of twofold nature; and on this being subdued, both

---

which retards the aspirant's spiritual growth. He used the word 'kamini,' or 'woman,' as a concrete term for the sex instinct when addressing his man devotees. He advised women, on the other hand, to shun 'man.' 'Kanchan,' or 'gold,' symbolizes greed, which is the other obstacle to spiritual life. Sri Ramakrishna never taught his disciples to hate any woman, or womankind in general. This can be seen clearly by going through all his teachings under this head and judging them collectively. The Master looked on all women as so many images of the Divine Mother of the Universe. He paid the highest homage to womankind by accepting a woman as his guide while practising the very profound spiritual disciplines of Tantra. His wife, known and revered as the Holy Mother, was his constant companion and first disciple. At the end of his spiritual practice he literally worshipped his wife as the embodiment of the Goddess Kali, the Divine Mother. After his passing away the Holy Mother became the spiritual guide not only of a large number of householders, but also of many monastic members of the Ramakrishna Order" (Swami Nikhilananda, trans., *The Gospel of Sri Ramakrishna* [New York: Ramakrishna-Vivekananda Center, 2000], 82).

the aforesaid five membered groups become subdued.... Never is desire appeased by the enjoyment of desires; it only waxes stronger, like fire [fed] by clarified butter.... These [organs], being contaminated with objects, are not capable of being subjugated by mere abstinence, as they are by ever present knowledge.... That man is to be known as having subjugated his sense-organs, who, on having heard, or touched, or seen, or tasted, or smelt, anything, neither rejoices nor grieves. From among all the organs, if one happens to ooze out, then thereby his wisdom oozes out, just like water from one part of the leathern bag. Having brought the host of organs under control, and having also subdued the mind, one should accomplish all his purposes, taking care not to injure his body.[55]

What are the dangers on the path of yoga?

The *Uddhava Gita* advises the spiritual seeker regarding the dangers of yoga practice:

Should the body of a Yogi, who is but practicing Yoga and is not yet adept in it, be overtaken by troubles that may have cropped up in the course of it, then the following remedies are prescribed.

Some evils [such as lust, etc.] he should slowly kill through meditation on Me [the Lord] and the chanting of My name, etc., and some [such as haughtiness, etc.] through service unto the great masters of Yoga.

There are some strong-willed people who by various means first make the body very strong and of undecaying youth, and then practice Yoga with a view to acquiring extraordinary powers.

But that is not praised by the wise, for such effort is useless, since the body is mortal, like the fruits of a tree [but the Atman is eternal].

If, in the course of regularly practicing Yoga, his body gets strong, the intelligent Yogi who is devoted to Me should not give up practice, pinning his faith on that. [He should not get attached to these powers, which are nothing in comparison with the majesty of the Atman.]

The Yogi who practices this Yoga, relying solely on Me and having no desires, is not thwarted by obstacles, and experiences the bliss of the Self.[56]

What are the benefits of *sattvika* living?

The *Uddhava Gita* mentions the following practices for increasing our *sattva* qualities:

The gunas sattva, rajas, and tamas belong to the intellect and not to the Self. Through sattva one should subdue the other two, and (subdue) sattva also by means of sattva itself. [One should control the functions of truthfulness, compassion, etc. through that absorption in Brahman.]

Through developed sattva a man attains to that form of spirituality which consists in devotion to Me [the Lord]. Through the use of sattvika things [i.e., those that tend to purity, illumination, and so on] sattva is developed; this leads to spirituality.

That superior form of spirituality which is brought on by an increase of sattva destroys rajas and tamas. And when both of these are destroyed, iniquity, which has its rise in them, is also quickly destroyed....

The fire that springs from the friction of bamboos in a forest burns that forest and is (itself) quenched. Similarly the body which is the outcome of an intermixture of the gunas is destroyed in the manner of the fire [i.e., the fire burns the whole forest by means of its flames; similarly the body destroys the gunas through knowledge manifested in it].[57]

Who is greater: the householder who lives in the world or the monk who has renounced everything for the sake of God?

There is a controversy regarding which is the highest goal of life: living in the world or embracing monastic life. The conventional view is that a monk is superior to the householder, but this view is not well founded. Regarding this question, Swami Vivekananda says:

> If a man retires from the world to worship God, he must not think that those who live in the world and work for the good of the world are not worshipping God. Neither must those who live in the world, working for the good of wife and children, think that those who give up the world are low vagabonds. Each is great in his own place. This thought I will illustrate by a story.
>
> A certain king used to inquire of all the sannyasins that came to his country, "Which is the greater man—he who gives up the world and becomes a sannyasin or he who lives in the world and performs his duties as a householder?" Many wise monks sought to solve the problem. Some asserted that the sannyasin was the greater, upon which the king demanded that they prove their assertion. When they could not do so, he ordered them to marry and become householders. Then others came and said, "The householder who performs his duties is the greater man." Of them, too, the king demanded proofs. When they could not give them, he made them also settle down as householders.
>
> At last there came a young sannyasin, and the king asked him the same question. He said, "Each, O King, is great in his own place." "Prove this to me," demanded the king. "I will prove it to you," said the sannyasin, "but you must come and live with me for a few days, that I may be able to prove to you what I say." The king consented. He followed the sannyasin

out of his own territory and they passed through many other countries until they came to a great kingdom. In the capital of that kingdom a ceremony was going on. The king and the sannyasin heard the noise of drums and music, and heard also the criers; the people were assembled in the streets in gala dress, and a proclamation was being made. The king and the sannyasin stood there to see what was going on. The crier was proclaiming loudly that the princess, the daughter of the king of that country, was about to choose a husband from among those assembled before her.

It was an old custom in India for princesses to choose husbands in this way. Each princess had certain ideas of the sort of man she wanted for a husband. Some wanted the handsomest man, others wanted only the most learned, others again the richest, and so on. All the princes of the neighbourhood would put on their best attire and present themselves before her. Sometimes they too had their own criers to enumerate their virtues—the reasons why they hoped the princess would choose them. The princess would be taken round on a throne, in the most splendid array, and would look at them and hear about them. If she was not pleased with what she saw and heard, she would say to her bearers, "Move on," and would take no more notice of the rejected suitor. If, however, the princess was pleased with any one of them, she would throw a garland of flowers over him and he became her husband.

The princess of the country to which our king and the sannyasin had come was having one of these interesting ceremonies. She was the most beautiful princess in the world, and her husband would be ruler of the kingdom after her father's death. The idea of this princess was to marry the handsomest man, but she could not find one to please her. Several such meetings had taken place, but the princess had been unable to select a husband. This meeting was the most splendid of all; more people than ever before attended it. The princess came in on a throne, and the bearers carried her from place to place. She did not seem to care for anyone, and everyone was disappointed, thinking that this meeting also was going to be a failure.

Just then a young man, a sannyasin, radiant as if the sun had come down to the earth, came and stood in one corner of the assembly, watching what was going on. The throne with the princess came near, and as soon as she saw the beautiful sannyasin, she stopped and threw the garland over him. The young sannyasin seized the garland and threw it off, exclaiming: "What nonsense is this? I am a sannyasin. What is marriage to me?" The king of that country thought that perhaps this man was poor and so dared not marry the princess, and said to him, "With my daughter goes half my kingdom now, and the whole kingdom after my death!" and put the garland on the sannyasin again. The young man threw it off once more, saying, "Nonsense! I do not want to marry," and walked quickly away from the assembly.

Now, the princess had fallen so much in love with this young man that she said, "I must marry this man or I shall die"; and she went after him to bring him back. Then our other sannyasin, who had brought the king there, said to him, "King, let us follow this pair." So they went after them, but at a good distance behind. The young sannyasin who had refused to marry the princess walked out into the country for several miles. When he came to a forest and entered it, the princess followed him, and the other two followed also. Now this young sannyasin was well acquainted with that forest and knew all the intricate paths in it. He suddenly entered one of these and disappeared, and the princess could not discover him. After vainly trying for a long time to find him, she sat down under a tree and began to weep, for she did not know the way out. Then our king and the other sannyasin came up to her and said: "Do not weep. We shall show you the way out of this forest, but it is too dark for us to find it now. Here is a big tree; let us rest under it, and in the morning we shall show you the road."

Now, a little bird and his wife and their three young ones lived in that tree, in a nest. This little bird looked down and saw the three people under the tree and said to his wife: "My dear, what shall we do? Here are some guests in the house, and it is winter, and we have no fire." So he flew away and got a bit of burning firewood in his beak and dropped it before the guests, to which they added fuel and made a blazing fire. But the little bird was not satisfied. He said again to his wife: "My wife, what shall we do? There is nothing to give these people to eat, and they are hungry. We are householders; it is our duty to feed anyone who comes to the house. I must do what I can; I will give them my body." So he plunged into the fire and perished. The guests saw him falling and tried to save him, but he was too quick for them.

The little bird's wife saw what her husband did, and she said: "Here are three persons and there is only one little bird for them to eat. It is not enough; it is my duty as a wife not to let my husband's effort go in vain. Let them have my body also." Then she fell into the fire and was burnt to death.

Then the three baby birds, when they saw what was done and that there was still not enough food for the three guests, said: "Our parents have done what they could and still it is not enough. It is our duty to carry on the work of our parents. Let our bodies go." And they too dashed down into the fire.

Amazed at what they saw, the three people could not of course eat these birds. They passed the night without food, and in the morning the king and the sannyasin showed the princess the way, and she went back to her father.

Then the sannyasin said to the king: "King, you have seen that each is great in his own place. If you want to live in the world, live like those birds, ready at any moment to sacrifice yourself for others. If you want to renounce the world, be like that young man, to whom the most beautiful woman and a kingdom were as nothing. If you want to be a householder, hold your life as a sacrifice for the welfare of others; and if you choose the life of renunciation, do not even look at beauty and money and power. Each is great in his own place, but the duty of the one is not the duty of the other."[58]

What are the duties of a householder and what are those of a monk?

Opinions differ with regard to the duties of householders and monks. Some maintain that there are not two religions—one for householders and another for monks. God-realization is the goal of life for both householders and monks. The required spiritual disciplines for God-realization are total renunciation, merciless dispassion, uncompromising self-control, and complete desire-lessness. Mastery of these virtues is vital not only for monks but also for householders. The scriptures make no concessions for householders.

There are others who say that a householder must practice internal renunciation, not external. *Sannyasa,* monastic life, is the fourth stage of life. The householder must fulfill the duties of a householder, first as a *brahmacharin* (celibate student), mastering both secular and sacred knowledge. Then the householder should enter family life, fulfill duties toward the family, earn money, and enjoy legitimate pleasures sanctioned by morality and ethics. Later, in the third stage, the householder should practice detachment from the family and spend more and more time in contemplation of God. Finally, in the fourth stage, the householder should follow the path of renunciation that is *sannyasa,* and walk alone.

The saying that one must renounce everything when the desire for such renunciation comes does not apply to householders. It would be utterly irresponsible for a householder to abandon family, children, father and mother, and take to the life of a *sannyasin* without making provisions for them. A person who ignores the duties of life as a householder is likely to ignore the duties of monastic life. Only a good householder can be a good monk. Through the performance of a householder's duties with nonattachment, a householder becomes ready for total renunciation for the sake of God.

Regarding the duties of a householder, Sri Ramakrishna says the following in conversations recorded in *The Gospel of Sri Ramakrishna*:

> *M.* (humbly): How ought we to live in the world?
>
> *Master:* Do all your duties, but keep your mind on God. Live with all—with wife and children, father and mother—and serve them. Treat them as if they were very dear to you, but know in your heart of hearts that they do not belong to you.
>
> A maidservant in the house of a rich man performs all the household duties, but her thoughts are fixed on her own home in her native village. She brings up her master's children as if they were her own. She even speaks of them as "my Rama" or "my Hari." But in her own mind she knows very well that they do not belong to her at all.
>
> The tortoise moves about in the water. But can you guess where her thoughts are? There on the bank, where her eggs are lying. Do all your duties in the world, but keep your mind on God.
>
> If you enter the world without first cultivating love for God, you will be entangled more and more. You will be overwhelmed with its danger, its grief, its sorrows. And the more you think of worldly things, the more you will be attached to them....
>
> But one must go into solitude to attain this divine love ... by meditating on God in solitude the mind acquires knowledge, dispassion, and devotion. But the very same mind goes downward if it dwells in the world.[59]

M: Sir, may I make an effort to earn more money?

Master: It is permissible to do so to maintain a religious family. You may try to increase your income, but in an honest way. The goal of life is not the earning of money, but the service of God. Money is not harmful if it is devoted to the service of God.

M: How long should a man feel obliged to do his duty toward his wife and children?

Master: As long as they feel pinched for food and clothing. But one need not take the responsibility of a son when he is able to support himself....[60]

[T]here is no hope for a worldly man if he is not sincerely devoted to God. But he has nothing to fear if he remains in the world after realizing God. Nor need a man have any fear whatever of the world if he attains sincere devotion by practicing spiritual discipline now and then in solitude. Chaitanya had several householders among his devotees, but they were householders in name only, for they lived unattached to the world.[61]

A Brahmo Devotee: Then, sir, we must give up our activities until we realize God?

Master: No. Why should you? You must engage in such activities as contemplation, singing His praises, and other daily devotions.

Brahmo: But what about our worldly duties—duties associated with our earning money, and so on?

Master: Yes, you can perform them too, but only as much as you need for your livelihood. At the same time, you must pray to God in solitude, with tears in your eyes, that you may be able to perform those duties in an unselfish manner. You should say to Him: "O God, make my worldly duties fewer and fewer; otherwise, O Lord, I find that I forget Thee when I am involved in too many activities. I may think I am doing unselfish work, but it turns out to be selfish."[62]

I tell you the truth: there is nothing wrong in your being in the world. But you must direct your mind toward God; otherwise you will not succeed. Do your duty with one hand and with the other hold to God. After the duty is over, you will hold to God with both hands....

Bondage is of the mind, and freedom is also of the mind. A man is free if he constantly thinks: "I am a free soul. How can I be bound, whether I live in the world or in the forest? I am a child of God, the King of Kings. Who can bind me?" ... By repeating with grit and determination, "I am not bound, I am free," one really becomes so—one really becomes free.[63]

What then is a man's duty? What else can it be? It is just to take refuge in God and to pray to Him with a yearning heart for His vision.[64]

Regarding the duties of a householder, Swami Vivekananda says:

The householder should be devoted to God; knowledge of God should be the goal of his life. Yet he must work constantly, perform all his duties; he must give up the fruits of his actions to God....

The great duty of the householder is to earn a living, but he must take care that he does not do it by telling lies or by cheating or by robbing others; and he must remember that his life is for the service of God and the poor.

Knowing that his mother and father are the visible representatives of God, the householder always and by all possible means must please them. If his mother is pleased, and his father, then God is pleased with that man. That child is really a good child who never speaks harsh words to his parents....

The mother and father are the causes of this body; so a man must undergo a thousand troubles in order to do good to them.

Even so is his duty to his wife. No man should scold his wife, and he must always maintain her as if she were his own mother. And even when he is in the greatest difficulties and troubles, he must not renounce his wife if she is chaste and devoted to him....

A son should be lovingly reared up to his fourth year; he should be educated till he is sixteen. When he is twenty years of age, he should be employed in some work; he should then be treated affectionately by his father as his equal. Exactly in the same manner the daughter should be brought up, and she should be educated with the greatest care....

Then there is the duty of a man towards his brothers and sisters, and towards the children of his brothers and sisters, if they are poor, and towards his other relatives, his friends, and his servants. Further, there are his duties towards the people of the same village, and the poor, and anyone that comes to him for help. If the householder, having sufficient means, does not care to help his relatives and the poor, know him to be only a brute; he is not a human being....

The householder is the center of life and society. It is a kind of worship for him to acquire and spend wealth nobly; for the householder who struggles to become rich by good means and for good purposes is doing practically the same thing for the attainment of salvation as the anchorite does in his cell when he prays; for in them we see only different aspects of the same virtue of self-surrender and self-sacrifice prompted by the feeling of devotion to God and to all that is His....[65]

Holy Mother Sri Sarada Devi's advice to householders is the following:

"Whenever you see a *sadhu,* you should show him respect. You should not show him disrespect by retorts or slighting remarks."

Regarding earning money and accumulating it, Mother said, "You have your wife and children. You should lay by something for them. What you have to consider, my boy, is that if you put by something, there will be some provision for your family and the future. Besides, you will be able to serve holy men too. If you have nothing, what will you give the holy men, my dear?

"My child, whatever one is, if he comes in the garb of a sannyasin, you do 'sadhu seva' (service to holy people) by offering him something or serving him in some way."

A disciple once asked, "The Master [Sri Ramakrishna] said that those who would accept him as their spiritual ideal would not be born again. Again Swamiji [Swami Vivekananda] said that no liberation is possible without being initiated into sannyasa. What, then, will be the way out for the householders?" To which the Mother responded, "Yes, what the Master said is true and what Swamiji said is also equally true. The householders have no need of external renunciation. They will spontaneously get internal renunciation. But some people need external renunciation. Why should you be afraid? Surrender yourself to the Master and always remember that he stands behind.

"Sri Ramakrishna used to say, 'One must practice self-control after the birth of one or two children.'"[66]

Regarding the duties of a monk (*sadhu*), Sri Ramakrishna says:

A sadhu should think of God with three quarters of his mind and with one quarter should do his other duties. He should be very alert about spiritual things. The snake is very sensitive in its tail. Its whole body reacts when it is hurt there. Similarly, the whole life of a sadhu is affected when his spirituality is touched.[67]

Sadhus should depend one hundred percent on God. They must not gather for the morrow.... Don't trust a sadhu if he keeps bag and baggage with him and a bundle of clothes with many knots. I have seen such sadhus under the banyan tree in the Panchavati. Two or three of them were seated there. One was picking over lentils, some were sewing their clothes, and all were gossiping about a feast they had enjoyed in a rich man's house. They said among themselves, "That rich man spent a hundred thousand rupees on the feast and fed the sadhus sumptuously with cake, sweets, and many such delicious things."[68]

[A] certain king ... gave a feast to the sadhus, using plates and tumblers of gold. I noticed in the monasteries of Benares with what great respect the abbots are treated. Many wealthy up-country people stood before them with folded hands, ready to obey their commands. But a true sadhu, a man who has really renounced everything, seeks neither a gold plate nor honour. God sees that he lacks nothing. God gives the devotee everything that is needed for realizing Him.[69]

Holy Mother says:

You [a monk] are a living god. Who is able to renounce all for God's sake? Even the injunctions of destiny are cancelled if one takes refuge in God. Destiny strikes off with her own hand what she has written about such a person.

The Master will be your protector. It will be a heinous sin on the part of the Master if he does not protect those who have taken shelter at his feet, who have taken refuge in him renouncing all, and who want to lead a good life. You must live in a spirit of self-surrender to him. Let him do good to you if he so desires, or let him drown you if that be his will. But you are to do only what is righteous, and that also according to the power he has given you.

A monk should be above attachment and jealousy.

A monk must sever all the chains of maya. Golden chains are as much of a bond as iron chains. A monk must have no attachments.

A monk should not visit his home. Meeting his people revives old memories. He must forget these, nay, his very body. Then only he can have a vision of God.

A monk may become very vain. He may think, "See, he does not respect me. He does not bow down before me," and so on.... Is it possible, my child, to get rid of vanity—vanity of beauty, vanity of virtue, vanity of knowledge, and vanity of a holy life?

It is the monk's duty to call on God. The monk cannot complain that God-vision is denied him in spite of hard struggle. God will reveal Himself at His will. He is not at anybody's beck and call.

To a woman disciple who was to lead an exclusive spiritual life, Holy Mother advised:

Never be intimate with any man—not even your own father or brother. What to speak of others then! Let me again repeat, don't be intimate with any man, even if God comes to you in that form.[70]

Swami Vivekananda says:

For the good of the many, for the happiness of the many, is the Sannyasin born. His life is all vain, indeed, who, embracing Sannyasa, forgets this ideal. The Sannyasin, verily, is born into this world to lay down his life for others, to stop the bitter cries of men, to wipe the tears of the widow, to bring peace to the soul of the bereaved mother, to equip the ignorant masses for the struggle for existence, to accomplish the secular and spiritual well-being of all through the diffusion of spiritual teachings and to arouse the sleeping lion of Brahman in all by throwing in the light of knowledge.

Getting the human birth, when the desire for Freedom becomes very strong, and along with it comes the grace of a person of realisation, then men's desire for Self-knowledge becomes intensified. Otherwise the mind of men given to lust and wealth never inclines that way. How should the desire to know Brahman arise in one who has the hankering in his mind for the pleasure of family-life, for wealth and for fame? He who is prepared to renounce all, who amid the strong current of the duality of good and evil, happiness and misery, is calm, steady, balanced, awake to his Ideal, alone endeavours to attain to Self-knowledge. He alone by the might of his own power tears asunder the net of the world ... one emerges like a lion, breaking the barriers of Maya.

One must have both internal and external Sannyasa—renunciation in spirit as well as formal renunciation.... Without dispassion for the world, without renunciation, without giving up the desire for enjoyment, absolutely nothing can be accomplished in the spiritual life.[71]

What is the significance of dreams?

Various interpretations of dreams have been given by different thinkers. It is a common belief that dreams foreshadow the future. Some hold that in the dream state, the dreamer goes out of the body. Aristotle believed the origin of dreams to be within the dreamer.

Aristotle no longer sought the origin of dreams outside man but inside his own nature. Dreams, he said, were the necessary manifestation of this nature. They derived from the experiences and personal attitudes of the dreamer, from his cares, his hopes, and also from his biological processes, especially from the coursing and warmth of blood. In his later writings he even tried to give a psycho-physiological explanation of prophetic dreams. However, the mere fact that he granted the possibility of prophetic dreams clearly proves that he too still based himself on the metaphysical foundations of the ancient Greeks.[72]

According to Freud, "all dreams are wish fulfillments" and are caused by infantile instincts.[73]

According to Vedanta, a dream is a dream; it does not have any spiritual validity. The emphasis of Vedanta is on the conscious mind and not on the subconscious. "Just as the physical and psychological aspect of an individual are inter-related, so are the three normal states of human experience—waking, dream, and dreamless sleep."[74] Analysis of any one of these states cannot give us the true meaning of dreams. Yet, a person's deep-seated tendencies or longings acquired by past karma in this life or previous lives can create dream imagery. Though, generally speaking, a person's secular disposition and desires give rise to dream images, there are cases when dreams indicate a dreamer's innate spiritual disposition.[75] Regarding this fact, Sri Ramakrishna says the following:

> [Sri Ramakrishna] asked a devotee, "Do you ever have dreams?"
>
> *Devotee:* Yes, sir. The other day I dreamt a strange dream. I saw the whole world enveloped in water. There was water on all sides. A few boats were visible, but suddenly huge waves appeared and sank them. I was about to board a ship with a few others, when we saw a brahmin walking over the expanse of water. I asked him, "How can you walk over the deep?" The brahmin said with a smile: "Oh, there is no difficulty about that. There is a bridge under the water." I said to him, "Where are you going?" "To Bhawanipur, the city of the Divine Mother," he replied. "Wait a little," I cried. "I shall accompany you."
>
> *Master:* Oh, I am thrilled to hear the story!
>
> *Devotee:* The brahmin said: "I am in a hurry. It will take you some time to get out of the boat. Good-bye. Remember this path and come after me."
>
> *Master:* Oh, my hair is standing on end! Please be initiated by a guru as soon as possible.[76]

When Holy Mother Sri Sarada Devi was asked, "Are dreams real?" Holy Mother said, "Yes, they are. Dreams regarding the Master are real, but he forbade his disciples to narrate, even to him, dreams regarding himself.... One may see a vision in a dream, but to see God in a physical form is a matter of rare good fortune."[77] Holy Mother once gave the following interpretation of a dream that was narrated to her:

> *Devotee:* Mother, I once dreamt that I was going to some place with my husband. We came to a river, the other bank of which could not be seen. We were going by the shady track along the river when a golden creeper so entwined my arms that I could not free them from it. From the other side of the river came a dark complexioned boy with a ferryboat. He said, "Cut off the creeper from your arm and then only will I take you across the river." I cut off almost the whole creeper but the last bit I could not get rid of. In the meantime my husband also disappeared. In despair I said to the boy, "I cannot get rid of this bit. You must take me to the other side." With these words I jumped into the boat. It sailed and my dream vanished.

> *Mother:* The boy whom you have seen is none other than Mahamaya, the great cosmic illusionist. She took you across the waters of the world in that form. Everything, husband, wife, or even the body, is only illusory. These are all shackles of illusion. Unless you can free yourself from these bondages, you will never be able to go to the other shore of the world. Even this attachment to the body, the identification of the self with the body, must go.[78]

What is the significance of astrological calculations?

Swami Saradananda says:

> The Master used to observe these things. He believed in auspicious and inauspicious times. And because he used to observe these things, we too observe them. But then, these calculations, nowadays, are not absolutely correct. There have been many changes in the position of the constellations and planets, but these astrological calculations have not been cor-

rected accordingly. So I do not observe them so much these days.[79]

What happens after death?

A disciple of Holy Mother once heard of a boy who was possessed by a ghost. Curious about the matter, he asked Holy Mother, "How long does one live in the spirit body?" To this, the Mother said:

All people, excepting highly evolved souls, live in the spirit body for a year. After that, food and water are offered in Gaya for the satisfaction of the departed souls and religious festivals are arranged. By these means the souls of the departed are released from their spirit body. They go to other planes of existence and experience pleasure or pain, and in course of time, are born again in human forms according to their desires. Others attain salvation from those planes. But if a person has some meritorious action to his credit in this life, he does not lose spiritual consciousness altogether in the spirit body.

The dialogue between the disciple and the Mother continued:

Disciple: Is it possible for one to attain to a higher state if one's sraddha ceremony [funeral rites] is performed in Gaya?

Mother: Yes, that is true.

Disciple: Then what is the necessity of spiritual practices?

Mother: These dead souls, no doubt, attain to a higher state and live there for some time, but afterwards they are again born in this world according to their past desires. After their birth in a human body, some of them obtain salvation in this life, whereas others take inferior births to reap the results of their karma. This world is moving around like a wheel. That indeed is the last birth in which one gets completely rid of all desires.

Disciple: You just referred to the dead souls attaining to a divine state. Do they go there by themselves or does someone lead them?

Mother: No, they go by themselves. The subtle body is like a body made of air.

Disciple: What happens to those for whom no sraddha ceremony is performed in Gaya?

Mother: They live in the spirit body until some fortunate ones born in their family perform the sraddha ceremony in Gaya or some other form of obsequies.

Disciple: We hear of ghosts and spooks. Are they the attendants of Siva or simply spirits? Or are they the spirits of dead people?

Mother: They are the spirits of the dead. The spirit attendants of Siva belong to a special group. One must live very carefully. Every action produces its results. It is not good to use harsh words towards others or be responsible for their suffering.[80]

Swami Saradananda mentions an incident that occurred at Kamarhati in 1885. Sri Ramakrishna and Swami Brahmananda were visiting the home of Gopala's mother and taking rest in the afternoon:

The Master [Sri Ramakrishna] saw a strange thing there at that time. We venture to state it here only because it was heard from the Master himself. Otherwise we would have suppressed it. The Master used to have only a little sleep during the whole of the day and night. He was therefore lying quiet. Rakhal [Swami Brahmananda] fell asleep by his side. The Master said, "A bad smell was felt. Then I saw two figures in a corner of the room. The appearance was hideous: Out of their bellies the entrails were hanging down and their faces, hands, and feet were exactly like the human skeletons arranged in the Medical College, which I saw at some time. They said to me humbly, 'Why are you here? Please go away from this place; we feel much pained (perhaps to remember their own condition) to see you.' On the one hand they were thus supplicating and, on the other, Rakhal was sleeping.

Seeing that they felt pained, I was going to get up and come away with my small bag and towel when Rakhal awoke and said, 'Where are you going?' Saying, 'I will tell you later on,' and catching hold of his hand, I came downstairs, and, taking leave of the old woman (she had just finished taking her food), I went and got into the boat. I then said to Rakhal, 'There are two ghosts there. The mill of Kamarhati is situated near the garden. They live in that room by smelling (for, with them, smelling is eating) the bones, etc., thrown away by the Europeans after they have taken their meal.' I said nothing of it to the old woman lest she should get afraid; for, she had always to live alone in that house."[81]

Regarding this encounter, a devotee asked Holy Mother, "Mother, those spirits must have been foolish. Instead of asking him for their liberation, they told him to go away." The Mother replied, "They will, no doubt, be liberated. His presence cannot be in vain. Once Naren (Swami Vivekananda) liberated a disembodied spirit in Madras."[82]

VARIOUS QUESTIONS TO SWAMI VIVEKANANDA AND HIS ANSWERS

The following are Swami Vivekananda's answers to a number of specific spiritual questions a disciple once asked the swami.

What is the controversy between knowledge and devotion?

The thing is, all this waging of war and controversy is concerning the preliminary ideals, i.e. those ideals which men take up to attain the real Jnana [Knowledge] or real Bhakti [Devotion]. But which do you think is the higher—the end or the means? Surely, the means can never be higher than the end, because the means to realise the same end must be numerous, as they vary according to the temperament or mental capacities of individual followers. The counting of beads, meditation, worship, offering oblations in the sacred fire—all these and such other things are the limbs of religion; they are but the means; and to attain to supreme devotion (Para-Bhakti) or to the highest realisation of Brahman is the pre-eminent end. If you look a little deeper, you will understand what they are fighting about. One says, "If you pray to God facing the East, then you will reach Him." "No," says another, "you have to sit facing the West, and then only will you see Him." Perhaps someone realised God in meditation, ages ago, by sitting with his face to the East, and his disciples at once began to preach this attitude, asserting that none can ever see God unless he assumes this position. Another party comes forward and inquires, "How is that? Such and such a person realised God while facing the West, and we have seen this ourselves." In this way all these sects originated. Some one might have attained supreme devotion by repeating the name of the Lord as Hari, and at once it entered into the composition of the Shastra as: "The name of the Lord Hari, the name of the Lord Hari alone. Verily, there is no other, no other, no other path than this in the age of Kali."

Someone, again, let us suppose, might have attained perfection with the name of Allah, and immediately another creed originated by him began to spread, and so on. But we have to see what is the end to which all these forms of worship and other religious practices are intended to lead. The end is shraddha. We have not any synonym in our Bengali language to express the Sanskrit word shraddha. The (Katha) Upanishad says that shraddha entered into the heart of Nachiketa. Even with the word *ekagrata* (one-pointedness) we cannot express the whole significance of the word shraddha. The word *ekagrata-nishtha* (one-pointed devotion) conveys, to a certain extent, the meaning of the word shraddha. If you meditate on any truth with steadfast devotion and concentration, you will see that the mind is more and more tending to Oneness, i.e. taking you towards the realisation of the absolute Existence-Knowledge-Bliss. The scriptures on Bhakti or Jnana give special advice to men to take up in life the one or the other of such nishthas (scrupulous persistence) and make it their own. With the lapse of ages, these great truths become distorted and gradually transform themselves into deshacharas, or the prevailing customs of a country. It has happened, not only in India, but in every nation and every society in the world. And the common people, lacking in discrimination, make these the bone of contention and fight among themselves. They have lost sight of the end, and hence sectarianism, quarrels, and fights continue.[83]

Should I practice meditation only in a worship room?

Those who have already realised the Lord's presence may not require it, but for others it is necessary. One, however, should go beyond the form and meditate on the impersonal aspect of God, for no form can grant liberation. You may get worldly prosperity from the sight of the form. One who ministers to his mother succeeds in this world; one who worships his father goes to heaven; but the worshipper of a sadhu (holy man) gets knowledge and devotion.[84]

What is the efficacy of prayer?

By prayer one's subtle powers are easily roused, and if consciously done, all desires may be fulfilled by it; but done unconsciously, one perhaps in ten is fulfilled. Such prayer, however, is selfish and should therefore be discarded.[85]

Where should I meditate—inside or outside the body? Should my mind be withdrawn inside or held outside?

We should try to meditate inside. As for the mind being here or there, it will take a long time before we reach the mental plane. Now our struggle is with the body. When one acquires a perfect steadiness in posture, then and then alone one begins to struggle with the mind. Asana (posture) being conquered, one's limbs remain motionless, and one can sit as long as one pleases.[86]

Sometimes I get tired of *japa*. Should I continue it?

One gets tired of japa for two reasons. Sometimes one's brain is fatigued, sometimes it is the result of idleness. If the former, then one should give up japa for the time being, for persistence in it at the time results in seeing hallucinations, or in lunacy etc. But if the latter, the mind should be forced to continue japa.[87]

When sitting for *japa*, I sometimes experience joy. But then I feel disinclined to continue the *japa* owing to that joy. Should I continue it then?

Yes, that joy is a hindrance to spiritual practice, its name being rasasvadana (tasting of the sweetness). One must rise above that.[88]

Should I practice *japa* even if my mind wanders?

Yes. As a person breaks a wild horse by always keeping his seat on its back.[89]

Should I control my emotions during meditation?

Meditate everyday alone. Everything will open up of itself. Now the Divine Mother—the embodiment of illumination—is sleeping within, hence you do not understand this. She is the Kundalini. When before meditation, you proceed to "purify the nerves," you must mentally strike hard on the Kundalini in the Muladhara (sacral plexus), and repeat, "Arise, Mother, arise!" One must practise these slowly. During meditation, suppress the emotional side altogether. That is a great source of danger. Those that are very emotional, have no doubt their Kundalini rushing quickly upwards, but it is as quick to come down as to go up. And when it does come down, it leaves the devotee in a state of utter ruin. It is for this reason that *kirtanas* and other auxiliaries to emotional development have a great drawback. It is true that by dancing and jumping etc., through a momentary impulse, that power is made to course upwards, but it is never enduring. On the contrary when it traces back its course, it rouses violent lust in the individual. Listening to my lectures in America, through temporary excitement many among the audience used to get into an ecstatic state, and some would even become motionless like statues. But on enquiry I afterwards found that many of them had an excess of the carnal instinct immediately after that state. But this happens simply owing to a lack of steady practice in meditation and concentration.[90]

Which spiritual ideal should I follow?

You have to make the character of Mahavira [Hanuman] your ideal. See how at the command of Ramachandra he crossed the ocean! He had no care for life or death! He was a perfect master of his senses and wonderfully sagacious. You have now to build your life on this great ideal of personal service. Through that all the other ideals will gradually manifest in life. Obedience to the guru without questioning, and strict observance of *brahmacharya*—this is the secret of success. As on the one hand Hanuman represents the ideal of service, so on the other he represents leonine courage, striking the whole world with awe. He has not the least hesitation in sacrificing his life for the good of Rama. A supreme indifference to everything except the service of Rama, even to the attainment of the status of Brahmā and Shiva, the great World-Gods! Only the carrying out of Sri Rama's behest is the one vow of his life!

Such whole-hearted devotion is wanted. Playing on the *khol* and *kartal* [earthen drum and cymbals] and dancing in the frenzy of *kirtana* has degenerated the whole people. They are, in the first place, a race of dyspeptics—and if in addition to this they dance and jump in that way, how can they bear the strain? In trying to imitate the highest *sadhana,* the preliminary qualification for which is absolute purity, they have been swallowed in dire *tamas.* In every district and village you may visit, you will find only the sound of the *khol* and *kartal*! Are not drums made in the country? Are not trumpets and kettledrums available in India? Make the boys hear the deep-toned sound of these instruments.... The *damaru* [an hour-glass-shaped drum] and horn have to be sounded, drums are to be beaten so as to raise the deep and martial notes and with "Mahavira, Mahavira" on our lips and shouting "Hara, Hara, Vyom, Vyom," the quarters are to be reverberated. The music which awakens only the softer feelings of man is to be stopped now for some time. Stopping the light tunes such as *kheal* and *tappa* [soft music] for some time, the people are to be accustomed to hear the *dhrupad* [deep] music. Through the thunder-roll of the dignified Vedic hymns, life is to be brought back into the country. In everything the austere spirit of the heroic manhood is to be revived. In following such an ideal lies the good of the people and the country. If you can build your character after such an ideal, then a thousand others will follow. But take care that you do not swerve an inch from the ideal. Never lose heart. In eating, dressing, or lying, in singing or playing, in enjoyment or disease, always manifest the highest moral courage. Then only will you attain the grace of Mahashakti, the Divine Mother.[91]

12

Lessons of History

$\mathcal{S}$ elf-knowledge or God-realization is the ultimate goal of life, and the yoga way teaches us that the rise or fall of an individual or a culture depends upon the attainment or neglect of spiritual wisdom. The spiritual goal of Self-knowledge alone makes all other human goals meaningful. But when we ignore the Self, our true identity, we face the same Self as the merciless law of history.

DIFFERENT VIEWS OF HISTORY

According to some worldviews, history is a meaningless venture. It is a story that carries no message, follows no logic, and serves no purpose. But this is an extreme view. If history were meaningless, life would be a product of natural necessity and a human individual an insignificant speck in the universe.

History is not just a narrative of events. It is a unique unfolding of certain facts that makes us reflect on our destiny. The proper study of humankind is the study of human history—our ideals and aspirations, hope and despair, achievements and failures. But, then, what is the precise nature of the goal toward which history moves? Are we on the path of progress? Is there any pattern or order that we can determine in the universe? Interpretations of history may be categorized as the following:

The providential view

The idealistic view

The linear view

The pluralistic view

The ethical and moral view

The cyclical view

The providential view

According to the providential view, history reveals a divine purpose. This view was formulated by the early Hebrews and by Christians. It was upheld by St. Augustine and the medieval church. History, according to this view, moves toward divine fulfillment. The will of God rules all history and God reveals his will through lawgivers and prophets.

In the beginning, God created heaven and earth, the first man and woman. Evil entered the world only when they disobeyed the command of God. Thus, human life is the scene of a constant struggle between the powers of good and evil. Since human beings are always vulnerable to sin and death, God sends messengers and prophets to guide them in the path of virtue and righteousness. History is the tension between God's will and the will of human beings. Life on earth is a preparation for the age of righteousness to come. There is an inherent disharmony between God's will and human will.

History, according to St. Augustine, is a revelation of God's will. There are two dispensations, side by side, in the world. The divine dispensation is for those who are predestined to be saved and the earthly dispensation for the unrighteous. History, therefore, is the arena of eternal conflict between two ideals, two sets of values, and two dispensations. It is the story of the fall and redemption of the human individual.

The idealistic view

The major author of the idealistic view of history is Hegel. The historical process, according to Hegel, is a dialectic movement in which civilization moves from nature to society and from the realm of law to the realm of freedom. The meaning of history is to be understood in the context of the state, because the state is the expressed form of society through which all individuals achieve self-fulfillment. Progress depends on the changes of the state toward freedom and reason. According to Hegel, history began in Asia. The second epoch is marked by the achievements of Greece and Rome, followed by the epoch of Christianity, and completed in the freedom and spirit of reason in Western Europe. Hegel saw a rational method guiding history as the process of the self-development of Absolute Spirit.

The linear view

According to the linear view, there is no need for a First Cause to explain the eternal creative order and no empirical reason to postulate a supernatural reality—something beyond nature. Nature is self-creative, self-supporting, and self-conserving. The universe does not show any preordained plan or purpose, and it would be contradictory to think that some Absolute Reality manifests itself through creation and yet human beings still have free will. So, according to this view, history is the record of natural facts, figures, dates, and places. The course of history is linear. It moves in a straight line, and its goal is progress.

Faith in the linear view expresses itself in the laws of evolution; from instinct to intellect and reason; from the individual to the family, tribe, nation, society, and state. The laws of natural selection and survival of the fittest operate everywhere. The historical process reveals a steady increase in peace, justice, reason, and morality in our societies. It is also the progressive growth of freedom—from dogma and superstition to rational and scientific thinking. Following this progressive trend, political thought has evolved from autocracy to democracy.

But the idea of endless progress is self-contradictory. It is as if by education and training we could produce any number of Michelangelos and Einsteins. If progress means anything, it means continuous approximation toward the goal. The factual evidence contradicts the assumption that there exists a perpetual linear trend applicable to all humankind. To accept the idea of an unbroken linear trend is to deny the other external forces that act upon such a trend. The state exists for the individual. The inviolable sanctity and freedom of the spirit is the justification of the state. History focuses on the individual, because truth reveals itself in the heart of the individual. To ignore the individual for the sake of the state is to make the state an omnicompetent community—a mortal God. The idea of a society with no conflict of ideals, no clash of interests, and no difference of views among individuals, is a utopia. As Sorokin aptly observes:

> Every page of human history bears witness to wars undertaken in the firm conviction that they would "end war," "abolish despotism," "make the world safe for democracy," overcome injustice, eliminate misery, and the like. And we observe "Homo sapiens" still engrossed in this crazy quest. From this standpoint, the history of human progress is indeed a history of incurable human stupidity![1]

The pluralistic view

The advocates of the pluralistic view interpret history in terms of the growth and decay of many cultures. According to this view, there is no such thing as a continuous world history. Each culture passes through four distinct stages analogous to the stages in the life of a person. First, there is the stage of infancy, which is the period of settlement and stabilization; people live in the state of nature. The second stage is the period of maturity. The third is the beginning of the decline; this decline is characterized by the growth of commerce, cosmopolitanism, science, technology, and philosophy. This stage is also marked by the rise of skepticism and secularism. The last is the stage of decay; at this stage, introversion is replaced by extroversion, spirituality by utility, and we witness the rise of industrial culture and the growth of secularism. History, according to Spengler, is made up of many cultures and does not necessarily move in a straight line.

The ethical and moral view

According to the ethical view, progress is not attained automatically. It is to be attained through ethical regeneration. But there is an inverse relationship between material progress and the ethical and moral virtues of individuals. Material achievement exerts a powerful influence on people and has a degenerative influence on human society that can only be overcome by cultural changes through proper education in the democratic outlook of life and by a return to the state of nature.

But the moral view of history does not explain *how* to recover from moral degeneration; it only demands that we must. Morality, in and of itself, cannot be the goal of a society. The foundation of any morality is not strong enough to withstand the impact of a degenerating culture. The moral person, who constantly battles against evil and imperfection, ultimately breaks down. Morality and ethics are stages on the way to spiritual growth, which transcends them. Culture is a way of life as well as a view of life. One's *way* of life cannot change unless inspired by a new, distinct, and vigorous *view* of life.

THE CYCLICAL VIEW

Against the background of these diverse views and speculations, Vedanta postulates a cyclical view of history. It is interesting to observe that the cyclical view, as propounded by the Vedic thinkers, was shared to a certain extent by the early Greeks, Romans, Stoics, and Chinese. One finds the reflection of the Vedic view in the writings of Marcus Aurelius and Seneca who believed in the theory of world cycles, which was again introduced by Nietzsche and Spengler in modern times. The Vedanta view, however, is quite different from these versions of the theory of world cycles in its depth of meaning.

The Absolute and the relative

According to Vedanta, history can be seen from two perspectives: the Absolute, or transcendental, point of view and the relative point of view. From the transcendental point of view, Brahman as Pure Being is the only Reality. Brahman alone exists and is beyond all ideas of time, space, causality, and history. Brahman is Existence-Knowledge-Bliss Absolute, the one without a second. But, until we realize our oneness with Brahman, the world remains real for us. From the relative point of view, Vedanta accepts the reality of the universe and history, and history follows a cyclical pattern. This creative process of history is integral, beginningless, eternal, and moves in cycles of creation, preservation, and destruction.

Vedanta philosophers maintain that there is an inherent unity in the midst of the apparent diversities of the universe. The power behind the universe is Brahman and the power behind the human individual is Atman (Self or soul). Brahman and Atman are identical in essence. God is an infinite circle whose circumference is nowhere but whose center is everywhere. The lessons of history and of evolution should awaken the spiritual seeker to this fact. The identity of God and a human individual has been declared by the four Vedic statements: "I am Brahman,"[2] "That thou Art,"[3] "This Atman is Brahman,"[4] and "Consciousness is Brahman."[5] These statements are verifiable through valid reasoning and open to the personal experiences of a seeker.

According to Vedanta, the great lesson of history is that the infinite Self, free and immortal, behaves at times like a bound creature due to maya, or metaphysical ignorance. As discussed in earlier chapters, maya is the inscrutable power of Brahman. It is through maya that Brahman, the Pure Being, appears as the creator, human beings, and the universe. It is ignorance that makes us see the universe as separate from Brahman. Brahman is ever present in creation, not in part, but as the undivided whole. Brahman is the sole reality in every being. The real nature of a human being, therefore, is a fascinating mystery that overshadows all other mysteries of the universe.

Psychoanalysts look upon human beings as deluded by their unconscious and held together by the tensions of opposite forces and contradictory tendencies; physiologists see humans as physiological organisms governed by definite chemical and neurological systems; physicists see humans as material mechanisms, blindly obeying the laws of physics. But we refuse to be exhausted by all these various speculations. We are not just a bundle of actions and reactions in a given medium at a fixed period of time or a product of natural necessity. Life introduces something incalculable and purposeful amidst the laws of nature, and we all feel this instinctively.

Human beings are essentially subjects and not objects. We are more than individuals, more than the sum of our appearances. The truth about our real nature lies hidden in the inner recess of our heart. Each of us is a soul who uses the body and mind as instruments to gain experiences of this world. Our real personality is a cosmic personality—the personality of God. By overlooking this cosmic personality, we develop an isolated, egocentric consciousness and behave like spiritual atoms separate from Pure Being. We create solitary prisons for ourselves, condemning ourselves to live in a world of egotistic existence far away from the broad currents of universal life. We become driven by pain and pleasure, birth and death, virtue and vice, and other pairs of opposites. These pairs of opposites are the laws of polarity, of cause and effect, and they apply to all that is in the realm of maya. Such laws, however, cannot affect the soul, which is ever free and immortal. History, then, is a continuous struggle to regain a lost balance. The search for happiness and self-fulfillment is essentially a search for immortality, which is our inner nature and about which we are forgetful. Ignorance keeps the wheel of suffering, of life and death, going round and round. Only Self-knowledge can make us free.

Thus, the entire cosmos is an integral manifestation of Pure Spirit. Creation, human beings, and nature are not different from one another in their essence. There was no time when nature did not exist. The sum total of energy always remains the same. What the naturalists call creation is nothing but evolution of energy into name and form. Time, space, and causality belong to nature and not to the soul. Therefore, the universe always exists, either in potential or in manifested form. A Hindu prayer says, "The sun and the moon, the Lord created like the suns and moons of previous cycles."[6] God is the ever-active Providence, by whose power world cycles evolve out of chaos, are made to run for a time, and are again destroyed. In the beginning of a particular cycle of evolution, the entire world is covered up by dissolution as the result of primordial reabsorption into Brahman. The elements gradually emerge from the state of absorption, and this may be called the evolution of the particular order. In the state of absorption, Brahman and maya remain in equilibrium. The creative power of Brahman, the seed force of things, and the individual souls existing in their subtle bodies, all remain absorbed in Brahman. Evolution, therefore, is indicative of the disturbance in the temporary equilibrium.

In each cycle, there is a recurrence of the same material phenomena, and the same recurrences continue throughout eternity. No force can die; no energy can be annihilated. They go on changing until they return to the source. The universe, when looked at from the point of view of the Absolute, has no history or development. The idea of history applies to the phenomenal universe, which is the self-expression of Brahman, the Pure Being, under the conditions of time, space, and causation.

History and the idea of progress

According to the cyclical view, the phenomenal world is always a mixture of good and evil. Good and evil are not two different entities. The idea that evil will be gradually eliminated and good will ultimately prevail is a contradiction in terms. The very idea of good implies evil; the very idea of life implies death. One cannot be separated from the other. As we increase our happiness, we increase our unhappiness. That which brings happiness to one, brings misery to another. That which is good for one may prove to be evil for another. The sum total of happiness and unhappiness always remains the same throughout all time. There is, then, the idea of equilibrium. But true equilibrium, according to the cyclical view, can never be achieved in the world. Equilibrium is absolute non-differentiation, which is neither desirable nor possible, because differentiation is the very fabric of nature. Creation is a struggle to regain the lost balance of perfection. History is made of struggle, conflict, and competition. Therefore, according to the cyclical view, there is no such thing as real progress; there is only change. We live in a changing world but not necessarily a progressive one. This is also the verdict of history. The problems of the phenomenal world remain the same. Civilization after civilization has tried to solve the problem of unhappiness, has tried to make the world a better and happier place, but the problems still remain.

Science and technology, for example, have changed our outer lives. The inscrutable atom has disclosed its secrets. We can now prolong the average span of life and explore nearby planets. New discoveries in the field of genetics are revolutionizing our knowledge and understanding of life's diversity. Yet, spiritually we have not progressed much further than the cavemen. In the name of progress, we have only converted our arrow into a missile and our club into a nuclear warhead. The cruelties of the barbarians of history pale into insignificance beside the atrocities and violence of the modern era. An isolated act of murder often fills our mind with horror and indignation, but the killing of thousands today does not stir our conscience. Hegel, in a biting remark, once said, "We learn only from history that mankind learns nothing from history."[7] Our redemption, according to the Vedanta philosophers, lies not in a faraway heaven but in our own soul. The Upanishad says:

> When men shall roll up space (akasa) as if it were a piece of hide, then there will be an end of misery without one's cultivating the Knowledge of the Lord, who is without parts, without actions, tranquil, blameless, unattached, the supreme bridge to Immortality, and like a fire that has consumed all its fuel.[8]

"Just as it is never possible to roll up the akasa as one does a piece of hide, so it is utterly impossible to put an end to misery without Knowledge of the Lord."[9] The light of Self-knowledge must shine within us if we are not to lose ourselves in the conquest of material improvements while remaining insecure and fearful within.

The course of history

For Vedanta thinkers, there is no such thing as an ideal society or an ideal historical situation. The phenomenal world, plagued by various pairs of opposites, is comprised of three *gunas* or subtle modes of nature: *sattva* (spirituality), *rajas* (activity), and *tamas* (passivity). The *gunas* move together and are inseparable. The three are present in everything in the world in varying proportions. The nature of an object is determined by the predominance of a particular *guna*, while the other two remain there in a suppressed state. The *gunas* influence the nature of every individual. When *sattva* prevails, the light of knowledge shines through the doorways of the senses. When *rajas* prevails, a person is stirred by greed, passion, desire, and arrogance. Delusion, inertia, and indolence are the characteristic marks of the *tamasika* manifestation. The three *gunas* influence our sense of values, understanding, and way of life.

The theory of the *gunas* has its bearing in the division of ancient Hindu society into four castes: priests, warriors, traders and farmers, and laborers. The caste system in Hinduism was the law of spiritual economics and had nothing to do with the superiority or inferiority of a particular group. The Vedas compare the four castes to four important parts of the body of the Cosmic Person: head, arms, thighs, and feet. The priest represents the head, the warrior the arms, the trader the thighs, and the laborer the feet. These four groups together preserve the efficiency, equilibrium, and harmony of social life. The health and welfare of society depend on the harmonious cooperation of the four. No one can go without the others. Exploitation or suppression of one by the others brings disintegration of the whole society. Such division of society into different castes becomes rigid and oppressive when the ideal of the Cosmic Person is overlooked. The idea of privilege creeps in and is claimed on grounds of spiritual superiority, social leadership, wealth, and class interest. Yet this is what repeatedly happens in the world. Every organized society, the Vedic philosophers observe, is generally ruled by each group in succession. Each enjoys power for a certain length of time and, again being corrupted by that power, yields place to the next group. This change of leadership in a society from one group to the other follows a cyclical pattern. Swami Vivekananda focuses our attention on this fact of cyclical change of leadership and its meaning:

> Each state has its glories as well as its defects. When the priest (brahmin) rules, there is a tremendous exclusiveness on hereditary grounds. The persons of the priests and their descendants are hemmed in with all sorts of safeguards. None

but they have any knowledge—none but they have the right to impart that knowledge. The glory of the priestly rule is that at this period is laid the foundation of the sciences. The priests cultivate the mind, for through the intellect they govern.

The military (kshattriya) rule is tyrannical and cruel, but not exclusive, and during that period the arts and social culture attain their height.

The commercial (vaisya) rule comes next. It is awful in its silent, crushing, blood-sucking power. Its advantage is that as the trader himself goes everywhere, he is a great disseminator of ideas collected during the two previous states. It is still less exclusive than the military, but culture begins to decay.

Last will come the labourer (sudra) rule. Its advantage will be the distribution of physical comforts; its disadvantage (perhaps) the lowering of culture. There will be a great distribution of ordinary education, but extraordinary geniuses will be fewer and fewer.

If it is possible to form a state in which the knowledge of the priest period, the culture of the military, the distributive spirit of the commercial, and the ideal of equality of the last can all be kept intact, minus their evils, it will be an ideal state. Is it possible?

Yet, the first three have had their time. Now is the time for the last—the sudras must have it—none can resist....

The other systems have been tried and found wanting. Let this one be tried—if for nothing else, for the novelty of the thing. A redistribution of pain and pleasure is better than always the same persons having pain or pleasure. The sum total of good and evil in the world remains ever the same. The yoke will be lifted from shoulder to shoulder by new systems—that is all.

Let every dog have his day in this miserable world, so that after this experience of so-called happiness they may all come to the Lord and give up this vanity of a world and governments and all other botherations.[10]

History and the goal of life

The cyclical view of Vedanta asserts the potential divinity of all human individuals and looks upon history not as a mechanical process of evolution but as the manifestation of divinity already within us. In a world plagued by competition, division, and suspicion, it teaches cooperation and solidarity. The Vedanta spiritual interpretation of human beings and our cosmos makes history meaningful in both its purpose and process. By conceiving of God as the center of all, it spiritualizes all historical events and situations.

The observation of the cyclical view is that God is both the efficient and material cause of the universe and that the world is an eternal stage of history, where God wears different masks of different human personalities and plays diverse roles on the human stage. In such an interpretation of history, every moment is a revelation.

Whether for the Phoenician trader, the Roman soldier, the Vedic seer, or the modern scientist, the human situation remains the same. History is the same quest for self-fulfillment, following diverse paths, ideologies, and socio-political systems. It is the same story of love and hatred, peace and war, pain and pleasure. The settings of history change, but the principles remain the same. When we look upon a particular event of history, it appears to be unique and unrepeatable. But when we look to the motivation behind each event, we find that history does in fact proceed cyclically.

The Vedanta view advocates neither pessimism nor optimism. While it is the attitude of a fool to be optimistic about everything, it is the attitude of a coward to despair of the events of history. The cyclical theory believes in the human individual—not the biological species or humanity in abstraction, but a particular individual—who takes a stand regardless of the absurdities of the relative world. Vedanta does not deny the world. It only says that it is not enough for human beings to cherish the idea of a unity that is small and frail. We must seek the true spiritual unity of the world and ourselves, which is an everlasting unity in Brahman.

The critics say that the cyclical view encourages asceticism, mysticism, and otherworldliness. But, then, all philosophy ends in spirituality. Without a spiritual goal, philosophy is nothing but talk about talk. Spirituality is not otherworldliness. Those whom we know to be the true friends of humanity are not naturalists or pragmatists but mystics. Theirs is the integral vision that unites the separate, elevates the base, purifies the impure, and ennobles the ignoble. A mystic is a universal personality, running against the current of popular prejudices, riding above the ignorance of the majority, and facing and overcoming the real problems of life.

Asceticism is not an anti-social, morbid view of life, or a life of sterile and monotonous existence. Asceticism is Self-assertion and Self-expansion. It is a stage through which every human being must pass. The true ascetic renounces the lower for the higher, the lesser for the greater. It is the positive force that fortifies every noble principle, strengthens every spiritual tradition, and sustains every great ideal. The spirit that is ready to suffer for the sake of truth alone can triumph over evil.

The lessons of history, the cyclical view claims, will remain undiscovered so long as we are preoccupied with the statistics of separate events. So long as we neglect the meaning of history, we lose the ontological sense, the sense of our organic relationship to Being. Maya, the mirage of Brahman, overwhelms us. We experience an eclipse of the soul. Under such circumstances, history proves to be no more than "a pack of tricks which we play upon the dead," as Voltaire asserted.[11] The crises of history are always the crises of values and spring from the crises of our souls. The recovery from such a crisis lies beyond history. It lies in realization of the Self.

We are threatened today by an all-engulfing crisis of history. Moral confusion, political conflict, and social unrest are only the outer symptoms of our inner crisis. This is the unique tragedy of modern times. But then, the Vedic thinkers say, we still have one unique gift. We can make our despair work for us. It is at the moment of despair that we hear the revelation of a truth that is beyond all history.

History, according to the Yoga and Vedanta view, teaches us that "When a civilization triumphs, it is more by the might of the spirit than by physical power. When it falls, it is through lack of spiritual vigour and vitality."[12] Civilizations and societies perish on account of spiritual bankruptcy. This same law determines the rise and fall of our individual lives. The rise of human individuals begins with their moral and spiritual rise, and the lack of morality and spirituality brings their downfall. This is the merciless law and lesson of history.

13
The Essential Teaching of Yoga

The philosophy of yoga tells us that the afflictions and tragedies of life are not due to the will of God, judgment of history, fate, luck, or chance, but due to our loss of contact with Ultimate Reality. This loss of contact is the root cause of our suffering, from which arise all secondary causes, such as fear, anxiety, pain, separation, attachment, and aversion.

According to yoga, Ultimate Reality is the Supreme Self, designated by various names as Purusha, Atman, Brahman, God, and Truth. The yoga way is the quest for the Self. This Self is the center of our being, the Consciousness of all consciousness, Goal of all goals, Support of all supports, and Reality of all realities. As the *Katha Upanishad* says:

> There is one Supreme Ruler, the inmost Self of all beings, who makes His one form manifold. Eternal happiness belongs to the wise, who perceive Him within themselves—not to others.[1]

Self-forgetfulness creates spiritual blindness that blocks or distorts our perception of Ultimate Reality. This Self-forgetfulness is the cause of all bondage and delusion. We forget our true Self due to ignorance. Ignorance first blocks the view of the Self and then projects a world that is illusory, impermanent, and imaginary. This world is plagued by the problems of change, suffering, uncertainty, and death. Material and psychological remedies do not and cannot help us overcome the problems of life. The yoga way contends that the problems of life, caused by the darkness of ignorance, can only be overcome by the light of Self-knowledge.

Self-knowledge alone overcomes death and guarantees our immortality. Immortality, according to yoga, is to be attained while living.[2] The *Katha Upanishad* reminds us:

> What is here, the same is there; and what is there, the same is here. He goes from death to death who sees any difference here.
>
> By the mind alone is Brahman to be realized; then one does not see in It any multiplicity whatsoever. He goes from death to death who sees multiplicity in It. This, verily, is That.[3]

One who dies in bondage will remain in bondage after death. One who does not attain peace here cannot expect peace hereafter.

Self-knowledge, according to yoga, is true liberation. A liberated soul sees all in the Self and the Self in all. Liberation does not merely mean goodness and piety but also wholeness, holiness, and self-expansion. It stands for increased integration, dynamic activity, all-embracing love, and untiring self-dedication. Only liberated souls demonstrate the reality of the Self and the knowledge of the Self. Self-knowledge is intense bliss, unrestricted awareness, and freedom from the apparently endless cycles of birth and death.

Knowledge of the Self is more than intellectual understanding and emotional exultation. Self-knowledge, according to yoga, is direct perception of Ultimate Reality, which calls for the rise of the whole mind and an intense longing for the Self. Such longing is preceded by a spiritual awakening that comes when we discover that nothing in this world can help us in our journey toward the Self and that nobody is there to save us from the terrors of life. This awakening is the fire of yoga that consumes all our false hopes and expectations. Yoga is also the light that illuminates everything within us and lets us perceive the reality of the Self within.

Direct perception of Reality calls for self-mastery, or control of the mind and the senses. The Self is like the bottom of a lake and the mind like the waters above. Due to countless waves of desires and temptations, the bottom of this lake remains unperceived. The disciplines of yoga aim at making the waters of this lake calm and tranquil. The essence of all disciplines is the cultivation of one single thought reminiscent of the Self, which is practiced through prayer, meditation, *japa,* or repetition of a sacred word, and austerities.

The yoga way assures us that the goal of spiritual quest is attainable, self-mastery possible, and liberation through Self-knowledge verifiable. When at last we realize oneness with our true Self within, we attain absolute freedom and unbounded joy. Liberation is the recovery of our soul from the bondage of a self-imposed ignorance. Life when not illumined by the light of Self-knowledge brings endless pain and suffering. But with knowledge of the Self, the liberated soul conquers death and becomes one with the Self in this very life. Liberation is the realization of what we have always been; it is regaining our true nature.

STEPS TO THE REALIZATION OF THE GOAL

The yoga way prescribes four values of life to attain Self-knowledge: dharma (righteousness), *artha* (wealth), *kama* (fulfillment of legitimate desires), and *moksha* (liberation of the soul).

Dharma is acting in accordance with our inner constitution. Dharma is formed by our past experiences and tendencies. It is the practice of righteous conduct in social life, which in turn helps us unfold the divinity within. *Artha* is the acquisition of that which is necessary for the preservation of our lives and the welfare of others. *Kama* is the fulfillment of legitimate pleasures, without which life becomes joyless and dry. *Moksha* is liberation of the

Self. Without this liberation, there is no peace, and without peace of mind, no duty is worth performing, no wealth worth acquiring, and no pleasure worth enjoying. Life is to be guided by all four basic values. Acquisition of wealth and enjoyment of sense pleasures are to be guided by righteousness (dharma) and governed by spiritual freedom (*moksha*).

The four values are normative concepts, which provide direction for our lives. *Moksha,* the supreme goal of life, is progressively achieved by following the path of gradual self-sublimation. The essential teaching of yoga is that we must spiritualize every aspect of our lives—not by suppressing our mind's natural expressions but by directing them to our true Self. All aspects of our lives must obey our dharma, which alone ensures the integrity of our social duties and individual freedom. Dharma is the conscious regulation of the gross urges toward the spiritual goal of Self-knowledge. Dharma endows us with physical fitness, mental strength, a moral foundation, and sound spiritual insight, ultimately preparing us for *moksha,* or spiritual illumination. All progress, according to yoga, is from the inner to the outer. One cannot see God unless one sees God within oneself.

Here, the question naturally arises: Why do we not see God who is self-evident and self-existent? Yoga answers: Because our mind is not pure. Only the pure mind can experience the pure Self. Moral purity is a prerequisite for practicing all spiritual discipline. But according to the way of yoga, spiritual discipline can never be standardized. The same cosmic Self resides in the hearts of all, but the inner disposition, body, mind, strength, natural ability, and desire for liberation are not the same in all seekers. Seekers therefore are generally described as active, emotional, scientific, or rational. The path of one may not be the path of another; but all sincere seekers attain the same goal of Self-knowledge or God-vision.

The yoga way prescribes four paths to Self-knowledge: the paths of selfless activity, divine love, concentration and meditation, and philosophical discrimination.

The yoga of selfless activity, or *karma-yoga,* is prescribed for those who are active by nature. It is not acting out of self-interest but selflessly serving God seated in the hearts of all. By this, the yogi of selfless action transforms every activity into a spiritual practice, a means for the attainment of ego-transcendence.

Those who are emotional by nature are asked to follow the yoga of divine love, or *bhakti-yoga.* For such persons, the formless, nameless, attributeless Ultimate Reality takes the form of a personal God. Seekers in this path direct all their emotions and love toward God and God alone. Yoga through love is the ceaseless adoration of absolute Reality.

The yoga of concentration and meditation, or *raja-yoga,* is for those who are by nature introspective and scientific. By their sheer strength of will and power of concentration, such seekers control the outward tendencies of the body in order to realize the one reality of the Self. This leads the seeker to *samadhi,* or transcendental realization. *Samadhi* is the birthright of us all. That which keeps us from attaining *samadhi* is nothing but our own restless minds. Mastery of the restless mind through ceaseless meditation on Ultimate Reality is the greatest practice of *raja-yoga.*

The yoga of philosophical discrimination, or *jnana-yoga,* is the path of self-analysis and complete renunciation. It is sacrificing all lesser goals, all temporary pleasures, and all earthly and heavenly rewards for the realization of the Self; for the Self "is dearer than wealth, dearer than son, and dearer than everything else, because it is Innermost," says the Upanishad.[4] *Jnana-yoga* is the direct path to knowledge of the Supreme Reality through discrimination, renunciation, self-control, and longing for liberation.

In brief, there is a veil of metaphysical ignorance that makes the mind think that it is separate from the Self. This veil must be gotten rid of—either by discovering its illusoriness with the insight of discriminatory knowledge (*jnana-yoga*), dissolving it in the ocean of divine love (*bhakti-yoga*), tearing it apart by the activity of selfless work (*karma-yoga*), or setting it on fire with the flames of meditation (*raja-yoga*). By any of these four methods, a person may overcome ignorance and attain infinite knowledge, unbounded awareness, and pure bliss.

The yoga way asserts that the conflicts and contradictions that shadow our everyday life can never be resolved by manipulating external nature. They cannot be resolved by intellectual rationalization. Even moral perfection cannot get rid of our suffering, whose root cause is spiritual. To resolve these conflicts we have to look to the bedrock of our existence and realize the Self.

The ultimate goal of life is to discover the divinity within ourselves and in all beings and things. This will lead us to adore our true Self, adore our fellow beings, and adore the world that is but a reflection of Reality. This reunion with the Absolute—the core of our individual being as well as of the universe—is the true meaning of yoga.

Yoga is the goal as well as the way of realistic living. Yoga seeks to transform us by raising our awareness of our true Self. Following the way of yoga, we move from the fever of desires to the serenity of desirelessness and from the illusion of bondage to the reality of freedom.

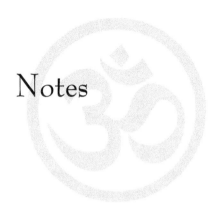

Notes

CHAPTER 1. THEORIES OF CREATION

1. See Chandradhar Sharma, *A Critical Survey of Indian Philosophy* (London: Rider & Company, 1960), 42.

2. Swami Nikhilananda, *Vivekananda: The Yogas and Other Works* (New York: Ramakrishna-Vivekananda Center, 1996), 87.

3. See Chandradhar Sharma, *Critical Survey of Indian Philosophy*, 55.

4. *Katha Upanishad* 1.2.1–2, in *The Upanishads*, vol. 1, trans. Swami Nikhilananda (New York: Ramakrishna-Vivekananda Center, 1990), 130–31.

5. Swami Madhavananda, trans., *Vivekachudamani of Sri Sankaracarya*, vv. 59–61 (Calcutta: Advaita Ashrama, 1970), 21–22.

6. *Gaudapada Karika* 2.34 of the *Mandukya Upanishad*, in *The Upanishads*, vol. 2, trans. Swami Nikhilananda (New York: Ramakrishna-Vivekananda Center, 2004), 275.

7. Ibid., 2.28, p. 268.

8. Ibid., 4.14–6, pp. 320–22.

9. Ibid., 2.32, p. 270.

10. S. Radhakrishnan, trans., *The Dhammapada* 170 (New York: Oxford University Press, 1968), 116.

11. Heraclitus frag. 14–16, in *Ancient Philosophy*, vol. 1 of *Philosophical Classics*, eds. Forest E. Baird and Walter Kaufmann (Englewood Cliffs, N.J.: Prentice Hall, 2000), 17.

12. See Chandradhar Sharma, *Critical Survey of Indian Philosophy*, 78.

13. Quoted in Satischandra Chatterjee and Dhirendramohan Datta, *An Introduction to Indian Philosophy* (Calcutta: University of Calcutta, 1948), 155.

14. See ibid., 73.

15. See ibid., 82.

16. See ibid., 189.

17. Quoted in ibid., 190.

18. Quoted in ibid., 190.

19. See Swami Adiswarananda, *The Vedanta Way to Peace and Happiness* (Woodstock, Vt.: SkyLight Paths Publishing, 2004), 31–32.

20. See Chandradhar Sharma, *Critical Survey of Indian Philosophy*, 165.

21. See ibid., 255.

22. See Swami Nikhilananda, *Bhagavad Gita* 4.1, p. 123.

23. Ibid., 10.8, p. 239.

24. Meister Eckhart, *Selected Writings*, trans. Oliver Davies (New York: Penguin Books, 1994), 10–11.

25. See Chandradhar Sharma, *Critical Survey of Indian Philosophy*, 346–48.

26. See ibid., 370.

27. See ibid., 368–69.

28. Swami Madhavananda, *Vivekachudamani*, v. 160, p. 61.

29. See Swami Nikhilananda, *Vivekananda: Yogas and Other Works*, 219–43.

30. Swami Madhavananda, *Vivekachudamani*, v. 539, p. 201.

31. Swami Madhavananda, *Vivekachudamani*, v. 542, p. 202.

32. S. Radhakrishnan, *Indian Philosophy*, vol. 2 (New York: The MacMillian Company, 1927), 659.

33. See P. Nagaraja Rao, *Introduction to Vedanta* (Bombay: Bharatiya Vidya Bhavan, 1958), 47.

34. See Chandradhar Sharma, *Critical Survey of Indian Philosophy*, 359.

35. See ibid., 279.

36. Quoted in ibid., 272.

37. See ibid., 157.

38. *Teachings of Sri Ramakrishna* (Calcutta: Advaita Ashrama, 1990), 5.

39. Swami Nikhilananda, *Vivekananda: Yogas and Other Works*, 531.

40. Ibid., 531.

Chapter 2. Sri Ramakrishna and the Thinkers of His Time

1. Swami Nikhilananda, trans., *The Gospel of Sri Ramakrishna* (New York: Ramakrishna-Vivekananda Center, 2000), 672.

2. Ibid., 649.

3. Ibid., 42.

4. Swami Saradananda, *Sri Ramakrishna, the Great Master*, trans. Swami Jagadananda (Madras: Sri Ramakrishna Math, 1970), 316.

5. Ibid., 316.

6. Swami Nikhilananda, *Gospel of Sri Ramakrishna*, 1010.

7. Ibid., 1020.

8. Ibid., 135.

9. Ibid., 318.

10. Ibid., 321.

11. Ibid., 1015.

12. Swami Saradananda, *Sri Ramakrishna, the Great Master*, 759.

13. Ibid., 689.

14. Ibid., 318.

15. Swami Nikhilananda, *Gospel of Sri Ramakrishna*, 236.

16. Ibid., 729.

17. Ibid., 650–51.

18. Ibid., 650.

19. Ibid., 158.

20. Swami Saradananda, *Sri Ramakrishna, the Great Master*, 696.

21. Ibid., 546.

22. Ibid., 696–97.

23. Swami Nikhilananda, *Gospel of Sri Ramakrishna*, 115–16.

24. Swami Saradananda, *Sri Ramakrishna, the Great Master*, 546–47.

25. Swami Nikhilananda, *Gospel of Sri Ramakrishna*, 99.

26. Ibid., 102.

27. Ibid., 888.

28. Ibid., 106, 108.

29. Ibid., 109.

30. Ibid., 267.

31. Ibid., 108.

32. Ibid., 669–70.

33. Ibid., 670.

34. Ibid., 672.

35. Ibid., 674.

36. Ibid., 675.

37. Swami Saradananda, *Sri Ramakrishna, the Great Master*, 845.

38. Ibid., 341.

39. Ibid., 341.

40. Ibid., 860.

41. Swami Nikhilananda, *Gospel of Sri Ramakrishna*, 916.

42. Ibid., 918.

43. Swami Saradananda, *Sri Ramakrishna, the Great Master*, 854.

44. Swami Nikhilananda, *Gospel of Sri Ramakrishna*, 853.

45. Ibid., 854–55.

46. Ibid., 867.

47. Ibid., 914–15.

48. Ibid., 884.

49. Ibid., 885.

50. Swami Saradananda, *Sri Ramakrishna, the Great Master*, 859.

51. Swami Nikhilananda, *Gospel of Sri Ramakrishna*, 852.

52. Ibid., 864.

53. Ibid., 879.

54. Ibid., 855.

55. Ibid., 910.

56. Swami Nikhilananda, *Vivekananda: Yogas and Other Works*, 183.

CHAPTER 3. SWAMI VIVEKANANDA: VEDANTA EAST AND WEST

1. Swami Nikhilananda, *Vivekananda: Yogas and Other Works*, 328.

2. Ibid., 375.

3. Ibid., 301.

4. Ibid., 267.

5. *Complete Works of Swami Vivekananda*, vol. 5 (Calcutta: Advaita Ashrama, 1970), 284–85.

6. Swami Nikhilananda, *Vivekananda: Yogas and Other Works*, 113.

7. Ibid., 113.

8. Ibid., 575.

9. R. C. Majumdar, ed., *Swami Vivekananda Centenary Memorial Volume* (Calcutta: Swami Vivekananda Centenary Committee, 1963), 187.

10. Ibid., 216–17.

11. Swami Vivekananda, *Thoughts of Power* (Calcutta: Advaita Ashrama, 1992), 13.

12. *Teachings of Swami Vivekananda* (Calcutta: Advaita Ashrama, 1971), 154.

13. R. C. Majumdar, *Swami Vivekananda Centenary Memorial Volume*, 213.

14. Ibid., 213.

15. Swami Nikhilananda, *Vivekananda: Yogas and Other Works*, 87.

16. Ibid., 929.

17. Ibid., 179.

CHAPTER 4. UNITY AND HARMONY OF RELIGIONS

1. Swami Nikhilananda, *Vivekananda: Yogas and Other Works*, 192–93.

CHAPTER 5. LOVE: HUMAN AND DIVINE

1. Swami Madhavananda, *Vivekachudamani*, v. 79, p. 29.

2. Ibid., v. 176, p. 68.

3. Swami Nikhilananda, *Gospel of Sri Ramakrishna*, 123.

4. *Brihadaranyaka Upanishad* 4.5.6, in *The Upanishads*, vol. 3, trans. Swami Nikhilananda (New York: Ramakrishna-Vivekananda Center, 1990), 309.

5. Erich Fromm, *The Art of Loving* (New York: Harper & Brothers Publishers, 1956), 26–29.

6. Swami Nikhilananda, *Gospel of Sri Ramakrishna*, 267.

7. Swami Nikhilananda, *Vivekananda: Yogas and Other Works*, 445–46.

8. Swami Nikhilananda, *Gospel of Sri Ramakrishna*, 942.

9. *Life of Sri Ramakrishna* (Calcutta: Advaita Ashrama, 1929), 667.

10. Swami Nikhilananda, *Holy Mother: Being the Life of Sri Sarada Devi, Wife of Sri Ramakrishna, and Helpmate in His Mission* (New York: Ramakrishna-Vivekananda Center, 1962), 134.

11. Swami Saradananda, *Sri Ramakrishna, the Great Master*, 794–95.

12. *Svetasvatara Upanishad* 3.16, in *Upanishads*, vol. 2, 103.
13. Swami Nikhilananda, *Gospel of Sri Ramakrishna*, 937.
14. Swami Nikhilananda, *Vivekananda: Yogas and Other Works*, 870, 872.
15. Swami Nikhilananda, trans., *Self-Knowledge* (New York: Ramakrishna-Vivekananda Center, 1989), 209.

CHAPTER 6. THE HUMAN MIND AND ITS HEALTH

1. Swami Nikhilananda, *Bhagavad Gita* 6.5–6, p. 163.
2. See Swami Nikhilananda, *Vivekananda: Yogas and Other Works*, 805–6.
3. Swami Madhavananda, trans., *Uddhava Gita or The Last Message of Sri Krishna* 8.4, 8.6 (Calcutta: Advaita Ashrama, 1971), 111–12.
4. Swami Nikhilananda, trans., *Bhagavad Gita* 5.23, p. 157.
5. *Sayings of Sri Ramakrishna* (Chennai: Sri Ramakrishna Math, 2003), 289.
6. Swami Nikhilananda, trans., *Bhagavad Gita* 6.34–35, p. 172.

CHAPTER 7. HUMAN RELATIONS: A SPIRITUAL GUIDE

1. Swami Nikhilananda, *Bhagavad Gita* 6.32, p. 171.
2. Ibid., 17.4–13, 17–22, pp. 333–37, 339–40.
3. Idib., 17.14–6, p. 338.
4. Shankaracharya, "A Cudgel for Delusion," v. 4, in Swami Nikhilananda, *Self-Knowledge*, 214.
5. *Talks with Swami Vivekananda* (Calcutta: Advaita Ashrama, 1946), 345
6. *Teachings of Sri Sarada Devi, the Holy Mother* (Madras: Sri Ramakrishna Math, 1983), 103.
7. Swami Nikhilananda, *Holy Mother*, 319.
8. Swami Nikhilananda, *Gospel of Sri Ramakrishna*, 86.
9. Swami Nikhilananda, trans., *The Gospel of Sri Ramakrishna*, abridged ed. (New York: Ramakrishna-Vivekananda Center, 1996), 133.
10. Ibid., 133.

CHAPTER 8. TRUTHFULNESS: ITS PRACTICE AND ITS DILEMMAS

1. Sissela Bok, *Lying: Moral Choice in Public and Private Life* (New York: Pantheon Books, 1978), xv, xvi.
2. Quoted in Sissela Bok, *Lying*, 32.

3. Ibid., 34.

4. Ibid, 73–74.

5. Swami Nikhilananda, *Gospel of Sri Ramakrishna*, 749.

6. Ibid., 176–77.

7. Ibid., 312.

8. *Complete Works of Swami Vivekananda*, vol. 6 (Calcutta: Advaita Ashrama, 1968), 124.

9. First Disciples of Shri Ramakrishna, *Spiritual Talks* (Calcutta: Advaita Ashrama, 1968), 268.

10. *Katha Upanishad* 2.2.13, in *The Upanishads*, vol. 1, 176.

11. *Mundaka Upanishad* 3.1.6, in *The Upanishads*, vol. 1, 300.

12. Swami Prabhavananda, *The Eternal Companion* (Hollywood: Vedanta Press, 1970), 271.

CHAPTER 9. THE TRUE FRIEND

1. Rick Weiss, "Aging—New Answers to Old Questions," in *National Geographic Magazine* 192, no. 5 (November 1997): 30.

2. *Complete Works of Swami Vivekananda*, vol. 4 (Calcutta: Advaita Ashrama, 1966), 366.

3. Quoted in Will Durant, *The Story of Philosophy* (New York: Garden City Publishing Co., Inc., 1926), 271.

4. Ralph Waldo Emerson, *Essays* (New York: Thomas Nelson and Sons, n.d.), 151.

5. Swami Nikhilananda, *Bhagavad Gita* 2.62–63, p. 96.

6. From *Narada Bhakti Sutras*, v. 44, quoted in Aswini Kumar Datta, *Bhaktiyoga* (Bombay: Bharatiya Vidya Bhavan, 1971), 34.

7. From *Narada Bhakti Sutras*, v. 45, quoted in ibid., 36.

8. Swami Madhavananda, *Uddhava Gita* 21.23, 26, pp. 317, 318.

9. *Complete Works of Swami Vivekananda*, vol. 8 (Calcutta: Advaita Ashrama, 1971), 83.

10. Swami Nikhilananda, trans., *The Gospel of Sri Ramakrishna* (New York: Ramakrishna-Vivekananda Center, 1992), 316.

11. Ibid., 609.

12. Swami Nikhilananda, *Bhagavad Gita* 2.40, p. 84.

CHAPTER 10. SIGNPOSTS OF PROGRESS

1. Swami Nikhilananda, *Bhagavad Gita* 6.31, p. 171.
2. Swami Nikhilananda, *Gospel of Sri Ramakrishna*, 404.
3. *Svetasvatara Upanishad* 2.11, in *Upanishads*, vol. 2, 93.
4. Swami Nikhilananda, *Gospel of Sri Ramakrishna*, 416.
5. Ibid., 503.
6. Ibid., 766.
7. Ibid., 624.
8. Swami Nikhilananda, *Vivekananda: Yogas and Other Works*, 609.
9. Swami Madhavananda, *Vivekachudamani*, v. 540, p. 201.
10. *Katha Upanishad* 1.2.23, in *The Upanishads*, vol. 1, 143.
11. Swami Nikhilananda, *Gospel of Sri Ramakrishna*, 497.
12. Ibid., 708.
13. Swami Nikhilananda, *Bhagavad Gita* 16.14–15, p. 328.
14. Swami Nikhilananda, *Gospel of Sri Ramakrishna*, abridged ed., 245–46, 368.
15. Ibid., 242.
16. Ibid., 126–27.
17. Swami Nikhilananda, *Bhagavad Gita*, 4.34, p. 141.

CHAPTER 11. VITAL SPIRITUAL QUESTIONS AND THEIR ANSWERS

1. Swami Nikhilananda, *Bhagavad Gita* 6.36, p. 173.
2. Ibid., 6.17, p. 167.
3. *Katha Upanishad* 2.3.11, in *The Upanishads*, vol. 1, 185.
4. Swami Nikhilananda, *Bhagavad Gita* 6.3, p. 162.
5. Swami Nikhilananda, *Gospel of Sri Ramakrishna*, 384.
6. Ibid., 542.
7. Ibid., 375.
8. Swami Nikhilananda, *Gospel of Sri Ramakrishna*, abridged ed., 312–13.
9. *Teachings of Sri Sarada Devi, the Holy Mother*, 141, 144–46, 147.
10. Swami Madhavananda, *Uddhava Gita*, v. 9.16, pp. 130–31.
11. Swami Nikhilananda, *Bhagavad Gita* 9.22, 6.40–42, 9.30–31, 9.26, pp. 174–75, 228, 230, 232.
12. Swami Nikhilananda, *Holy Mother*, 222.
13. Ibid., 220.

14. See M. P. Pandit, *Gems from the Tantras: Second Series* (Madras: Ganesh & Co. Private Ltd., 1970), 63.

15. See ibid., 67.

16. See ibid., 66.

17. *Teachings of Sri Sarada Devi, the Holy Mother*, 39, 50–51.

18. Swami Nikhilananda, *Holy Mother*, 151.

19. Swami Moksadananda, trans., *Jivan-Mukti-Viveka of Swami Vidyaranya* (Calcutta: Advaita Ashrama, 1996), 235–37.

20. Sri Swami Sivananda, *Dhyana Yoga* (Rishikesh: The Yoga Vedanta Forest University, 1958), 11.

21. Swami Chetanananda, trans., *A Guide to Spiritual Life: Spiritual Teachings of Swami Brahmananda* (St. Louis: Vedanta Society of St. Louis, 1988), 160.

22. Ibid., 160–61.

23. Ibid., 161.

24. Ganga-Natha Jha, trans., *Manu-Smriti: The Laws of Manu with the Bhasya of Medhatithi*, vol. 1, part 2, 220–21 (Calcutta: University of Calcutta, 1921), 514, 516.

25. Ibid., 516.

26. Swami Chetanananda, *A Guide to Spiritual Life*, 161–62.

27. Swami Nikhilananda, *Bhagavad Gita* 6.16, p. 166.

28. Swami Aseshananda, *Glimpses of a Great Soul: A Portrait of Swami Saradananda* (Portland, Ore.: Vedanta Society of Portland, 1982), 142–43.

29. Ibid., 197.

30. *Talks with Swami Vivekananda*, 249.

31. Swami Chetanananda, *A Guide to Spiritual Life*, 162.

32. Swami Aseshananda, *Glimpses of a Great Soul*, 199.

33. Swami Nikhilananda, *Self-Knowledge*, 171.

34. Ibid., 171–72.

35. Swami Madhavananda, *Vivekachudamani*, v. 6, p. 3.

36. Ibid., v. 56, pp. 20–21.

37. Ibid., vv. 418–24, pp. 158–60.

38. Swami Yatiswarananda, *The Adventures in Religious Life* (Madras: Sri Ramakrishna Math, n.d.), 310.

39. Ibid., 310–32

40. Ibid., 312–13.

41. Swami Nikhilananda, *Vivekananda: Yogas and Other Works*, 596–97.

42. *Complete Works of Swami Vivekananda*, vol. 5, 323.

43. Swami Nikhilananda, *Vivekananda: Yogas and Other Works*, 547–48.

44. M. P. Pandit, *Gems from the Tantras*, 46.

45. See ibid., 47.

46. Ganga-Natha Jha, *Manu-Smriti*, 521–27, 530, 535.

47. Ibid., 469, 472–74, 499–500.

48. See M. P. Pandit, *Gems from the Tantras*, 28.

49. First Disciples of Shri Ramakrishna, *Spiritual Talks*, 16–17.

50. *Complete Works of Swami Vivekananda*, vol. 5, 322.

51. Swami Nikhilananda, *Gospel of Sri Ramakrishna*, 401.

52. Ibid., 750.

53. Ibid., 112.

54. Ibid., 739.

55. Ganga-Natha Jha, *Manu-Smriti*, 354, 361–63.

56. Swami Madhavananda, *Uddhava Gita*, vv. 23.38–44, pp. 353–55.

57. Ibid., vv. 8.1–5, 7, pp. 110–13.

58. Swami Nikhilananda, *Vivekananda: Yogas and Other Works*, 468–70.

59. Swami Nikhilananda, *Gospel of Sri Ramakrishna*, 81–82.

60. Ibid., 114.

61. Ibid., 126.

62. Ibid., 142.

63. Ibid., 137–38.

64. Ibid., 671.

65. Swami Vivekananda, *Karma-Yoga and Bhakti-Yoga* (New York: Ramakrishna-Vivekananda Center, 1989), 20–25.

66. *Teachings of Sri Sarada Devi, the Holy Mother*, 6, 9, 11, 12, 15.

67. Swami Nikhilananda, *Gospel of Sri Ramakrishna*, 440.

68. Ibid., 314–15.

69. Ibid., 521.

70. *Teachings of Sri Sarada Devi, the Holy Mother*, 1, 25–28, 30, 33, 35, 38, 40.

71. *Teachings of Swami Vivekananda*, 250–51.

72. Swami Satprakashananda, *The Goal and the Way* (St. Louis: The Vedanta Society of St. Louis, 1977), 166.

73. Ibid., 167.

74. Ibid., 171.

75. Ibid., 164.

76. Swami Nikhilananda, *Gospel of Sri Ramakrishna*, 122–23.

77. Swami Nikhilananda, trans., Swami Adiswarananda, ed., *Sri Sarada Devi, The Holy Mother: Her Teachings and Conversations* (Woodstock, Vt.: SkyLight Paths Publishing, 2004), 191, 197.

78. Ibid., 95.

79. Swami Aseshananda, *Glimpses of a Great Soul*, 197.

80. Swami Nikhilananda and Swami Adiswarananda, *Sri Sarada Devi, The Holy Mother*, 140–41.

81. Swami Saradananda, *Sri Ramakrishna, the Great Master*, 663.

82. Swami Nikhilananda, trans., *Sri Sarada Devi, the Holy Mother, Book II: Her Conversations* (Madras: Sri Ramakrishna Math, 1980), 261.

83. *Complete Works of Swami Vivekananda*, vol. 5, 385–87.

84. Ibid., 323.

85. Ibid., 325.

86. Ibid., 324.

87. Ibid.

88. Ibid.

89. Ibid.

90. *Talks with Swami Vivekananda*, 307–8.

91. Ibid., 279–81.

CHAPTER 12. LESSONS OF HISTORY

1. P. A. Sorokin, *The Crisis of Our Age* (New York: E. P. Dutton & Co., Inc., 1942), 326.

2. *Brihadaranyaka Upanishad*, 1.4.10, in *The Upanishads*, vol. 3, 122–23.

3. *Chhandogya Upanishad*, 6.8.7, in *The Upanishads*, vol. 4, trans. Swami Nikhilananda (New York: Ramakrishna-Vivekananda Center, 1994), 309.

4. *Mandukya Upanishad*, v. 2, in *Upanishads*, vol. 2, 224.

5. *Aitareya Upanishad*, 3.1.3, in *The Upanishads*, vol. 3, 38–39.

6. See Swami Vimalananda, trans., *Mahanarayana Upanishad*, 1.64–65 (Madras: Sri Ramakrishna Math, 1979), 83.

7. Quoted in S. Radhakrishnan, *Kalki or the Future of Civilization* (New York: E. P. Dutton & Co., 1929), 53.

8. *Svetasvatara Upanishad*, 6.19–20, in *Upanishads*, vol. 2, 141–42.

9. See ibid., 141.

10. Swami Nikhilananda, *Vivekananda: Yogas and Other Works*, 922–23.

11. Quoted in Will Durant, *Story of Philosophy*, 241.

12. S. Radhakrishnan, *Kalki or the Future of Civilization*, 52.

CHAPTER 13. THE ESSENTIAL TEACHING OF YOGA

1. *Katha Upanishad*, 2.2.12, in *The Upanishads*, vol. 1, 175.

2. See Swami Nikhilananda, *Bhagavad Gita* 13.12, pp. 288–89.

3. *Katha Upanishad*, v. 2.1.10–1, in *The Upanishads*, vol. 1, 165–66.

4. *Brihadaranyaka Upanishad*, 1.4.8, in *The Upanishads*, vol. 3, 121.

Glossary

advaita Nonduality; a school of Vedanta philosophy declaring the oneness of God, soul, and universe.

anahata A sound that may be heard in meditation at a certain stage of spiritual unfoldment; the word is also applied to Om.

Atman Self or Soul; denotes also the Supreme Soul, which, according to the Advaita Vedanta, is one with the individual soul.

Avatar or Avatara Incarnation of God.

avidya Ignorance, cosmic or individual, which is responsible for the non-perception of Reality.

Bhagavad Gita An important Hindu scripture, part of the *Mahabharata* epic, containing the teachings of Sri Krishna.

bhakta A follower of the path of *bhakti*, divine love; a worshipper of the personal God.

bhakti Devotion; love of God.

bhakti-yoga The path of devotion followed by dualistic worshippers.

bhavasamadhi Ecstasy in which the devotee retains his or her ego and enjoys communion with the personal God.

Brahmā The creator god; the first person of the Hindu trinity, the other two being Vishnu and Siva.

brahmachari or *brahmacharin* A celibate student undergoing mental and moral training under a preceptor in the old Hindu style; a novice in a Hindu monastery preparing for the life of a monk.

brahmacharya The state of a brahmachari; the life of an unmarried student.

Brahman The Absolute; the Supreme Reality.

brahmana Same as brahmin.

Brahmananda, Swami A sannyasin disciple of Sri Ramakrishna, also known by the pre-monastic name of Rakhal.

brahmin The highest caste in Hindu society.

Chaitanya, Sri A prophet born in 1485, who lived at Navadip, Bengal, and emphasized the path of divine love for the realization of God.

Dakshineswar The suburb of Calcutta wherein is situated the Kali temple of Rani Rasmani, in which Sri Ramakrishna stayed for the greater part of his life.

daya Compassion.

guna One of the basic modifications of nature. According to the Samkhya philosophy, Prakriti (Nature), in contrast with Purusha (Spirit), consists of three *gunas* (qualities or strands), known as *sattva, rajas,* and *tamas.*

Hari God; a name of Vishnu.

hatha yoga A school of yoga that chiefly aims at physical health and well-being.

Holy Mother See Sarada Devi, Sri.

Ishta or Ishtadevata The form or an aspect of the deity one specially selects for devotional purposes; Chosen Ideal.

japa or *japam* Silent repetition of a divine name or a mystic syllable, keeping count either with a rosary or fingers. This kind of repetition occupies an important place in the Hindu system of spiritual practice.

jiva The embodied soul; a living being; an ordinary person.

jivanmukti Liberation from maya while living in the body.

jnana Knowledge of God arrived at through reasoning and discrimination; also denotes the process of reasoning by which the ultimate truth is attained. The word is generally used to denote the knowledge by which one is aware of one's identity with Brahman.

jnana-yoga Spiritual discipline mainly based upon philosophical discrimination between the real and the unreal, and renunciation of the unreal.

jnani One who follows the path of knowledge, consisting of discrimination to realize God; generally used to denote a non-dualist.

Kali An epithet of the Divine Mother, the Primal Energy.

Kaliyuga See *yuga*.

Kalpataru The Wish-fulfilling Tree; refers to God.

karma (1) Action in general; duty. (2) The law of cause and effect.

karma-yoga Spiritual discipline based upon the unselfish performance of duty without attachment to the fruits of action.

Krishna, Sri A divine incarnation, described in the *Mahabharata* and *Bhagavatam*.

kundalini The spiritual energy lying coiled up, or dormant, at the base of the spine in all individuals. When awakened through spiritual practice, it rises through the spinal column, passes through various centers, *chakras,* and at last reaches the brain, whereupon the yogi experiences *samadhi.*

lila Divine sport or play. Creation is often explained by the Vaishnavas as the spontaneous *lila* of God.

M. Mahendra Nath Gupta, the author of *The Gospel of Sri Ramakrishna* and a prominent householder disciple of Sri Ramakrishna.

Mahabharata A celebrated Hindu epic.

mantra or mantram A sacred word or mystic syllable in Sanskrit, used in *japa.*

Manu The ancient Hindu lawgiver.

Master, the An honorific name for Sri Ramakrishna.

maya Ignorance obscuring the vision of God; the Cosmic Illusion on account of which the One appears as many, the Absolute as the relative; it is also used to denote attachment.

Mimamsa One of the six systems of orthodox Hindu philosophy.

mukti Liberation from the bondage of the world, which is the goal of spiritual practice.

Nag Mahashay A householder disciple of Sri Ramakrishna.

Naren or **Narendra** See **Vivekananda, Swami.**

Nirguna Brahman Brahman without qualities or attributes.

nirvikalpa samadhi The highest state of *samadhi,* in which the aspirant realizes his total oneness with Brahman.

Nyaya Indian Logic, one of the six systems of orthodox Hindu philosophy.

Om The most sacred word of the Vedas; a symbol of God and of Brahman.

paramahamsa One belonging to the highest order of *sannyasis.*

Patanjali The author of the Yoga system, one of the six systems of orthodox Hindu philosophy.

Prakriti Primordial Nature, which, in association with Purusha, creates the universe. It is one of the categories of the Samkhya philosophy.

prarabdha **karma** The action that has begun to fructify, the fruit of which is being reaped in this life.

Puranas Books of Hindu mythology.

Purusha A term of the Samkhya philosophy, denoting the eternal Conscious Principle; the universe evolves from the union of Prakriti and Purusha. The word also denotes the soul and the Absolute.

rajas The principle of activity or restlessness. See *guna.*

rajasika Pertaining to, or possessed of, *rajas.*

raja-yoga A system of Yoga ascribed to Patanjali, dealing with concentration and its methods, control of the mind, *samadhi,* and similar matters.

Rama or **Ramachandra, Sri** The hero of the *Ramayana,* regarded by the Hindus as a Divine Incarnation.

Ramakrishna, Sri (1836–1886) A great saint of Bengal, regarded as a divine Incarnation, whose life inspired the modern renaissance of Vedanta.

sadhana Spiritual discipline.

sadhu Holy personality; a term generally used with reference to a monk.

Saguna Brahman Brahman with attributes and qualities; the Absolute conceived as the creator, preserver, or destroyer of the universe; the personal God, according to Vedanta.

samadhi Total absorption in the object of meditation or in the Godhead; ecstasy.

Samkhya One of the six systems of orthodox Hindu philosophy.

samskara A tendency, habit, predisposition, or mental impression created by thoughts and actions.

sannyasa Monastic life.

sannyasin A monk.

Sarada Devi, Sri (1853–1920) Wife and spiritual companion of Sri Ramakrishna; also known as the Holy Mother.

Saradananda, Swami (1865–1927) A monastic disciple of Sri Ramakrishna.

sattva The principle of balance or wisdom. See *guna.*

sattvika Pertaining to, or possessed of, *sattva.*

savikalpa samadhi In Vedanta, the first of two stages of *samadhi,* in which the seeker remains conscious of his realization of the unity of his inmost self with the Supreme Self.

Shankaracharya (788–820) One of the greatest philosophers of India, an exponent of Advaita Vedanta.

shraddha Faith.

siddhi Spiritual attainment acquired through practice of yoga.

sishya Disciple.

Sri (also Shri) Literally, "blessed" or "holy." A prefix used with names or the titles of certain scriptures. It serves as an honorific title before the name of a deity or holy man or woman.

tamas The principle of inertia or dullness. See *guna.*

tamasika Pertaining to, or possessed of, *tamas*.

Tantra A system of religious philosophy in which the Divine Mother, or Power, is the Ultimate Reality; also the scriptures dealing with this philosophy.

tapas or *tapasya* Austerity.

Uddhava Gita A text that forms part of the *Shrimad Bhagavatam*. It is the parting instructions of Sri Krishna to his beloved devotee and follower Uddhava.

Upanishads Scriptures that contain the inner or mystic teachings of the Vedas, dealing with the ultimate Truth and its realization.

Vaisesika One of the six systems of orthodox Hindu philosophy.

Vaishnava Lit., follower of Vishnu. A member of the well-known dualistic sect of that name, generally the followers of Sri Chaitanya in Bengal and of Ramanuja and Madhva in south India.

Vedanta One of the six systems of orthodox Hindu philosophy.

Vedas The revealed scriptures of the Hindus, consisting of the *Rig Veda, Sama Veda, Yajur Veda,* and *Atharva Veda*.

Vivekananda, Swami (1863–1902) The foremost of Sri Ramakrishna's *sannyasin* disciples, known also by the pre-monastic name of Narendra, or by the still shorter term, Naren.

Vrindavan A town on the bank of the Jamuna River associated with Sri Krishna's childhood.

Yoga (1) One of the six systems of orthodox Hindu philosophy. The Yoga system of Patanjali. (2) Union of the individual soul with the Universal Soul. (3) The method by which to realize union through control of mind and concentration.

yuga A cycle or world period. According to Hindu mythology, the duration of the world is divided into four *yugas,* namely, Satya, Treta, Dwarapa, and Kali. In the first, also known as the Golden Age, there is a preponderance of virtue among human beings, but with each succeeding *yuga,* virtue diminishes and vice increases. In the Kaliyuga there is a minimum of virtue and an excess of vice. The world is said to be now passing through the Kaliyuga.

Credits

Grateful acknowledgment is given for permission to use material from the following sources:

From *Uddhava Gita or The Last Message of Sri Krishna* translated by Swami Madhavananda, 1971; *Complete Works of Swami Vivekananda*, vol. 8, 1971; *Complete Works of Swami Vivekananda*, vol. 5, 1970; *Talks with Swami Vivekananda*, 1939; *Spiritual Talks* by the First Disciples of Shri Ramakrishna, 1968; *Vivekachudamani of Sri Sankaracarya* translated by Swami Madhavananda, 1970; "Swami Vivekananda: His Message of Vedanta and the Western Way" by Swami Adiswarananda from *Prabudha Bharata*, 1995, used by permission of the publisher, Advaita Ashrama, Calcutta, West Bengal, India.

From *A Guide to Spiritual Life: Spiritual Teachings of Swami Brahmananda* translated by Swami Chetanananda, © 1988, used by permission of the publisher, Vedanta Society of St. Louis.

From *Sri Ramakrishna, the Great Master* by Swami Saradananda, translated by Swami Jagadananda, 1970; *Teachings of Sri Sarada Devi, the Holy Mother*, 1983; "The Message of Unity and Harmony of Religions" by Swami Adiswarananda from *The Vedanta Kesari*, 1995, used by permission of the publisher, Sri Ramakrishna Math, Chennai, India.

About the Author

Swami Adiswarananda, a senior monk of the Ramakrishna Order of India, is the Minister and Spiritual Leader of the Ramakrishna-Vivekananda Center of New York. Born in 1925 in West Bengal, India, Swami received his undergraduate and Master's degrees from the University of Calcutta. He joined the monastic order of Sri Ramakrishna in 1954 and was ordained a monk in 1963. Before being sent by the Ramakrishna Order to its New York center in 1968, he taught religious subjects in one of the premier colleges of the Order and was later editor of *Prabuddha Bharata: Awakened India*, the English-language monthly journal on religion and philosophy published by the Order. Swami is a frequent lecturer at colleges, universities, and other religious, educational, and cultural institutions, and his writings appear regularly in many scholarly journals on religion and philosophy. He is the author of *The Vedanta Way to Peace and Happiness* and *Meditation and Its Practices: A Definitive Guide to Techniques and Traditions of Meditation in Yoga and Vedanta* (both SkyLight Paths). He is also the editor of *Sri Ramakrishna, the Face of Silence* and *Sri Sarada Devi, The Holy Mother: Her Teachings and Conversations* (both SkyLight Paths).

About SKYLIGHT PATHS Publishing

SkyLight Paths Publishing is creating a place where people of different spiritual traditions come together for challenge and inspiration, a place where we can help each other understand the mystery that lies at the heart of our existence.

Through spirituality, our religious beliefs are increasingly becoming a part of our lives—rather than *apart* from our lives. While many of us may be more interested than ever in spiritual growth, we may be less firmly planted in traditional religion. Yet, we do want to deepen our relationship to the sacred, to learn from our own as well as from other faith traditions, and to practice in new ways.

SkyLight Paths sees both believers and seekers as a community that increasingly transcends traditional boundaries of religion and denomination—people wanting to learn from each other, *walking together, finding the way.*

For your information and convenience, at the back of this book we have provided a list of other SkyLight Paths books you might find interesting and useful. They cover the following subjects:

Buddhism / Zen	Gnosticism	Mysticism
Catholicism	Hinduism /	Poetry
Children's Books	Vedanta	Prayer
Christianity	Inspiration	Religious Etiquette
Comparative	Islam / Sufism	Retirement
Religion	Judaism / Kabbalah /	Spiritual Biography
Current Events	Enneagram	Spiritual Direction
Earth-Based	Meditation	Spirituality
Spirituality	Midrash Fiction	Women's Interest
Global Spiritual	Monasticism	Worship
Perspectives		

Or phone, mail or e-mail to: SKYLIGHT PATHS Publishing
An imprint of Turner Publishing Company
4507 Charlotte Avenue • Suite 100 • Nashville, Tennessee 37209
Tel: (615) 255-2665 • www.skylightpaths.com
Prices subject to change.

Sacred Texts—SkyLight Illuminations Series
Andrew Harvey, series editor

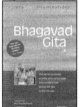

Offers today's spiritual seeker an enjoyable entry into the great classic texts of the world's spiritual traditions. Each classic is presented in an accessible translation, with facing pages of guided commentary from experts, giving you the keys you need to understand the history, context, and meaning of the text. This series enables readers of all backgrounds to experience and understand classic spiritual texts directly, and to make them a part of their lives. Andrew Harvey writes the foreword to each volume, an insightful, personal introduction to each classic.

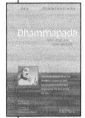

Bhagavad Gita: Annotated & Explained
Translation by Shri Purohit Swami; Annotation by Kendra Crossen Burroughs
"The very best Gita for first-time readers." —Ken Wilber. Millions of people turn daily to India's most beloved holy book, whose universal appeal has made it popular with non-Hindus and Hindus alike. This edition introduces you to the characters, explains references and philosophical terms, shares the interpretations of famous spiritual leaders and scholars, and more.
5½ x 8½, 192 pp, Quality PB, ISBN 1-893361-28-4 **$16.95**

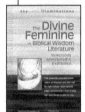

Dhammapada: Annotated & Explained
Translation by Max Müller and revised by Jack Maguire; Annotation by Jack Maguire
The Dhammapada—believed to have been spoken by the Buddha himself over 2,500 years ago—contain most of Buddhism's central teachings. This timeless text concisely and inspirationally portrays the route a person travels as he or she advances toward enlightenment and describes the fundamental role of mental conditioning in making us who we are.
5½ x 8½, 160 pp, b/w photographs, Quality PB, ISBN 1-893361-42-X **$14.95**

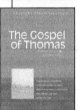

The Divine Feminine in Biblical Wisdom Literature
Selections Annotated & Explained
Translation and annotation by Rabbi Rami Shapiro; Foreword by Rev. Dr. Cynthia Bourgeault
Uses the Hebrew books of Psalms, Proverbs, Song of Songs, Ecclesiastes and Job, and the Wisdom literature books of Sirach and the Wisdom of Solomon to clarify who Wisdom is, what She teaches, and how Her words can help us live justly, wisely, and with compassion.
5½ x 8½, 240 pp, Quality PB, ISBN 1-59473-109-8 **$16.99**

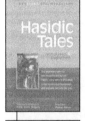

The Gospel of Thomas: Annotated & Explained
Translation and annotation by Stevan Davies
Discovered in 1945, this collection of aphoristic sayings sheds new light on the origins of Christianity and the intriguing figure of Jesus, portraying the Kingdom of God as a present fact about the world, rather than a future promise or future threat.
5½ x 8½, 192 pp, Quality PB, ISBN 1-893361-45-4 **$16.95**

Hasidic Tales: Annotated & Explained
Translation and annotation by Rabbi Rami Shapiro
Introduces the legendary tales of the impassioned Hasidic rabbis, which demonstrate the spiritual power of unabashed joy, offer lessons for leading a holy life, and remind us that the Divine can be found in the everyday.
5½ x 8½, 240 pp, Quality PB, ISBN 1-893361-86-1 **$16.95**

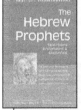

The Hebrew Prophets: Selections Annotated & Explained
Translation and annotation by Rabbi Rami Shapiro
Focuses on the central themes covered by all the Hebrew prophets: moving from ignorance to wisdom, injustice to justice, cruelty to compassion, and despair to joy, and challenges us to engage in justice, kindness, and humility in every aspect of our lives.
5½ x 8½, 224 pp, Quality PB, ISBN 1-59473-037-7 **$16.99**

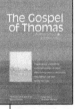

Sacred Texts—SkyLight Illuminations Series
Andrew Harvey, series editor

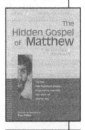

The Hidden Gospel of Matthew: Annotated & Explained
Translation and annotation by Ron Miller
Takes you deep into the text cherished around the world to discover the words and events that have the strongest connection to the historical Jesus. Reveals the underlying story of Matthew, a story that transcends the traditional theme of an atoning death and focuses instead on Jesus's radical call for personal transformation and social change.
5½ x 8½, 272 pp, Quality PB, ISBN 1-59473-038-5 **$16.99**

The Secret Book of John
The Gnostic Gospel—Annotated & Explained
Translation and annotation by Stevan Davies

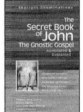

Introduces the most significant and influential text of the ancient Gnostic religion. This central myth of Gnosticism tells the story of how God fell from perfect Oneness to imprisonment in the material world, and how by knowing our divine nature and our divine origins—that we are one with God—we reverse God's descent and find our salvation.
5½ x 8½, 208 pp, Quality PB, ISBN 1-59473-082-2 **$16.99**

Rumi and Islam: Selections from His Stories, Poems, and Discourses—Annotated & Explained
Translation and annotation by Ibrahim Gamard

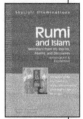

Offers a new way of thinking about Rumi's poetry. Focuses on Rumi's place within the Sufi tradition of Islam, providing insight into the mystical side of the religion—one that has love of God at its core and sublime wisdom teachings as its pathways.
5½ x 8½, 240 pp, Quality PB, ISBN 1-59473-002-4 **$15.99**

Selections from the Gospel of Sri Ramakrishna
Annotated & Explained
Translation by Swami Nikhilananda; Annotation by Kendra Crossen Burroughs

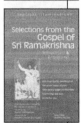

The words of India's greatest example of God-consciousness and mystical ecstasy in recent history. Introduces the fascinating world of the Indian mystic and the universal appeal of his message that has inspired millions of devotees for more than a century.
5½ x 8½, 240 pp, b/w photographs, Quality PB, ISBN 1-893361-46-2 **$16.95**

The Way of a Pilgrim: Annotated & Explained
Translation and annotation by Gleb Pokrovsky

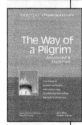

This classic of Russian spirituality is the delightful account of one man who sets out to learn the prayer of the heart—also known as the "Jesus prayer"—and how the practice transforms his life.
5½ x 8½, 160 pp, Illus., Quality PB, ISBN 1-893361-31-4 **$14.95**

Zohar: Annotated & Explained
Translation and annotation by Daniel C. Matt

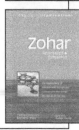

The best-selling author of *The Essential Kabbalah* brings together in one place the most important teachings of the Zohar, the canonical text of Jewish mystical tradition. Guides you step by step through the midrash, mystical fantasy, and Hebrew scripture that make up the Zohar, explaining the inner meanings in facing-page commentary.
5½ x 8½, 176 pp, Quality PB, ISBN 1-893361-51-9 **$15.99**

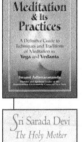

Global Spiritual Perspectives

Spiritual Perspectives on America's Role as Superpower
by the Editors at SkyLight Paths

Are we the world's good neighbor or a global bully? Explores broader issues surrounding the use of American power around the world, including in Iraq and the Middle East. From a spiritual perspective, what are America's responsibilities as the only remaining superpower? Contributors:

Dr. Beatrice Bruteau • Rev. Dr. Joan Brown Campbell • Tony Campolo • Rev. Forrest Church • Lama Surya Das • Matthew Fox • Kabir Helminski • Thich Nhat Hanh • Eboo Patel • Abbot M. Basil Pennington, ocso • Dennis Prager • Rosemary Radford Ruether • Wayne Teasdale • Rev. William McD. Tully • Rabbi Arthur Waskow • John Wilson

5½ x 8½, 256 pp, Quality PB, ISBN 1-893361-81-0 **$16.95**

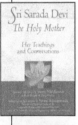

Spiritual Perspectives on Globalization, 2nd Edition
Making Sense of Economic and Cultural Upheaval
by Ira Rifkin; Foreword by Dr. David Little, Harvard Divinity School

What is globalization? What are spiritually minded people saying and doing about it? This lucid introduction surveys the religious landscape, explaining in clear and nonjudgmental language the beliefs that motivate spiritual leaders, activists, theologians, academics, and others involved on all sides of the issue. This edition includes a new Afterword and Discussion Guide designed for group use.

5½ x 8½, 256 pp, Quality PB, ISBN 1-59473-045-8 **$16.99**

Hinduism / Vedanta

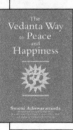

Meditation & Its Practices: A Definitive Guide to Techniques and Traditions of Meditation in Yoga and Vedanta
by Swami Adiswarananda

The complete sourcebook for exploring Hinduism's two most time-honored traditions of meditation. Drawing on both classic and contemporary sources, this comprehensive sourcebook outlines the scientific, psychological, and spiritual elements of Yoga and Vedanta meditation.

6 x 9, 504 pp, HC, ISBN 1-893361-83-7 **$34.95**

Sri Sarada Devi: Her Teachings and Conversations
Translated and with Notes by Swami Nikhilananda
Edited and with an Introduction by Swami Adiswarananda

Brings to life the Holy Mother's teachings on human affliction, self-control, and peace in ways both personal and profound, and illuminates her role as the power, scripture, joy, and guiding spirit of the Ramakrishna Order.

6 x 9, 288 pp, HC, ISBN 1-59473-070-9 **$29.99**

The Vedanta Way to Peace and Happiness
by Swami Adiswarananda

Using language that is accessible to people of all faiths and backgrounds, this book introduces the timeless teachings of Vedanta—divinity of the individual soul, unity of all existence, and oneness with the Divine—ancient wisdom as relevant to human happiness today as it was thousands of years ago.

6 x 9, 240 pp, HC, ISBN 1-59473-034-2 **$29.99**

Or phone, mail or e-mail to: SKYLIGHT PATHS Publishing
An imprint of Turner Publishing Company
4507 Charlotte Avenue • Suite 100 • Nashville, Tennessee 37209
Tel: (615) 255-2665 • www.skylightpaths.com
Prices subject to change.

Printed in the USA
CPSIA information can be obtained
at www.ICGtesting.com
JSHW022213140824
68134JS00018B/1035

9 781683 364412